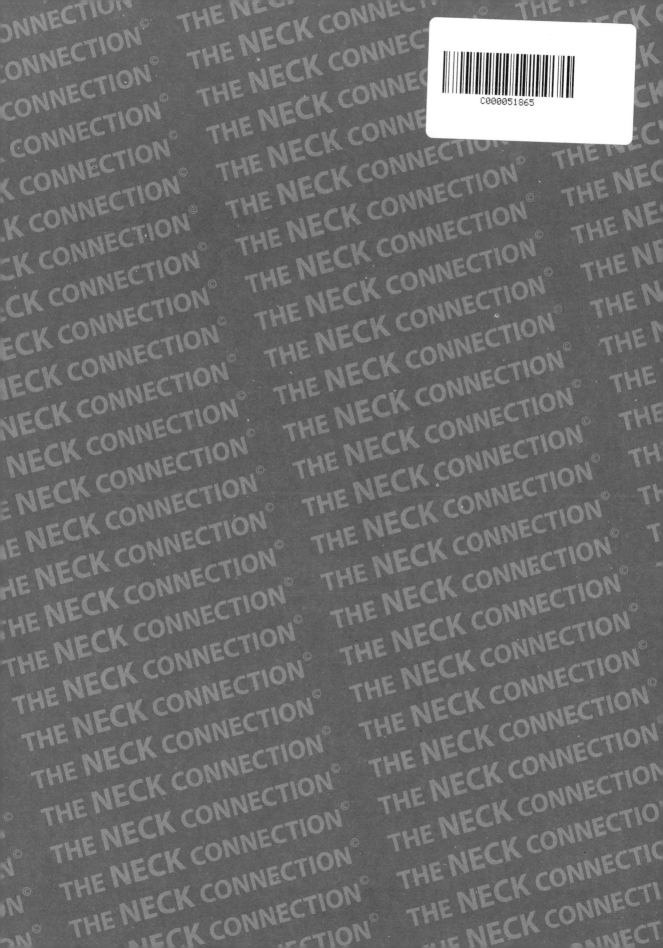

About Dr. Mosaraf Ali

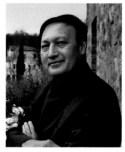

Dr. Mosaraf Ali is a pioneer in integrated medicine. He blends the science of conventional medicine with elements of traditional systems such as herbal medicine, Ayurveda and Unani to produce a unique, safe and highly effective method of healthcare. His philosophy is based on the Hippocratic Principles, which state that we all have an innate healing power that can cure most ailments and restore wellbeing. Dr Ali's simple lifestyle programme of diet, massage, yoga and natural supplements nurtures this healing power. It has been developed over 28 years of clinical experience, working with patients from all walks of life, from the most disadvantaged to celebrities and royalty.

Dr Ali has written seven books and wrote a health column for six years in The Mail on Sunday and in Top Santé magazine. He trains doctors in integrated medicine, has carried out research into the effects of his massage therapy in stroke rehabilitation, speaks regularly at conferences around the world and heads the clinical spa at Castel Monastero in Tuscany, Italy, as well as practising from his central London clinic. He also has a charity clinic in a village in the Indian Himalayas, providing free medical care to over 50,000 needy people.

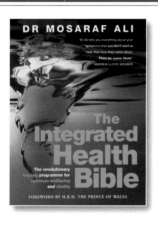

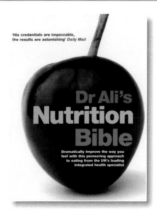

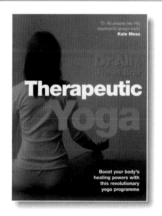

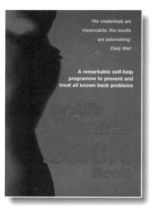

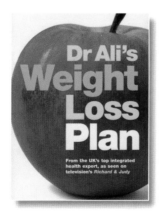

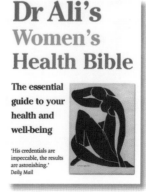

To
His Majesty
Sultan Qaboos
Bin Said Al Said,

The Sultanate of Oman

First Published in Great Britain 2011

Published by Integrated Health Products Ltd. (Integrated Medical Center)
121 Crawford Street, London, United Kingdom, W1U 6BE.
Telephone: +44 207 2245 111
Email: info@theneckconnection.com
Website: www.drmali.com

Printed and bound by:
Paragraphics
D-222, Abul Fazal Enclave, Jamia Nagar, New Delhi-110025, India

Edited by Ken Bridgewater

ISBN 09569028-0-1

CONTENTS

PART 2

PART 3

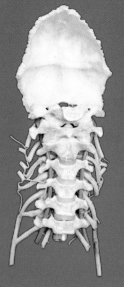

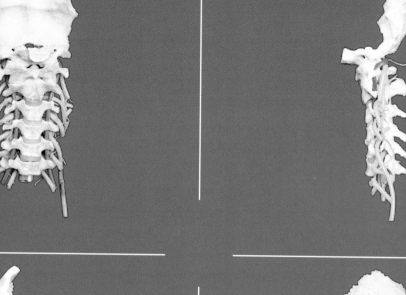

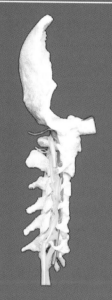

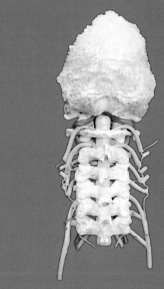

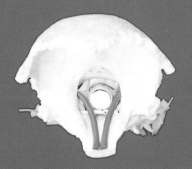

Actual Photos of the

location of the

Vertebral Arteries

in the Neck & Inside the Skull

(feeding the brain)

The Neck Connection ©

Dr Mosaraf Ali

The Subconscious Brain is a little understood part of our being, yet it is responsible for controlling practically every aspect of our lives. Using the subconscious brain we live, emote, reproduce, digest, protect ourselves, heal and regulate all our bodily functions. We also react to external stimuli, sleep, wake, make love, coordinate, stand, carry out skills, eat, maintain homoeostasis (constant body temperature, maintenance and blood parameters). All of these, and more, use the subconscious brain. This book reveals my discovery and hypothesis, that the uncontrollable part of the involuntary brain *can be* controlled and influenced to function more efficiently by improving the blood supply to it. The more nutrition, oxygen, glucose, micro elements etc. you supply to it through blood and brain fluid, the better those functions will be carried out.

The basic logic is that the conscious brain appeared much later in the evolution of the brain and is therefore present in mammals. On the other hand reptiles, amphibians, birds, fish and insects still only have the involuntary or automatic brain functioning on its own or with instinct without a conscious command. The two parts of the brain have two separate circulatory networks. In strict principle, the carotid artery, which is located in the front of the neck, hidden behind the firmer muscles, predominantly supplies blood to the conscious or voluntary brain. That is the part that thinks, makes decisions, has logic, deduces, analyses, sees colours or shapes, hears and stores sounds, or words, in our long-term memory and gives us intelligence. How quickly and effectively we carry out these functions depends largely on this supply. It cannot for example, help in the process of digestion, hormonal regulation, body temperature control or improve the immune system. These are highly complicated processes. The vertebral arteries and veins, however, are located in a canal, formed by the bodies of the neck vertebrae and thick fibrous sheaths. The body has taken utmost care in protecting these blood vessels. I discovered that these are vital

INTRODUCTION

because they nourish the most crucial and delicate parts of the brain known as The Subconscious Brain.   Eureka! For centuries, it was an accepted belief, especially in India, that you need to meditate, sublimate, eat vegetarian food, control your thoughts and relate them to the subconscious brain.

After years of perseverance devotees were able to slow down their breathing and heart rate. They were able to go into a "near death" state of "Samadhi" or deep hibernation, influence healing, even cure diseases. This book illustrates how you can influence your well-being, health, mental and bodily functions simply by improving blood flow to the very part of the brain that regulates all these.

You need to learn a little anatomy to know how these blood vessels are affected by accidents, traumas, stress, birth injuries, posture or surgeries sustained in the neck area. The fragile and delicately balanced cervical vertebrae dislocate or misalign at their joints and compress or twist these vital arteries in the process. That reduces blood supply to the subconscious brain and alters its normal vital functions. Correct the faults with my unique technique of therapy with massage, manipulation, specific yoga exercises and change in diet and `bingo', you automatically heal and normal functions of the body are restored.

This is the simple solution to very complicated questions: why are we ill and why do we function under par? And what we can do about it, is the revolutionary idea detailed in this book.

I have worked unceasingly to prove my hypotheses for more than 20 years, against all odds, facing challenges and criticism. I have carried out my therapy on thousands of patients, to deduce, formulate, and ascertain the Neck Connection in Disease and Health.

This is my seventh book. As an established writer, speaker and doctor I have pioneered integrated medicine in specific fields and I want to share the contents of this book with you. I hope my discovery is further researched and put to use to understand and treat numerous diseases to help mankind relieve itself of discomfort and suffering.

PART 1

The Problem

The Revelation

Traditionally a sharp blow to the neck can be fatal. No other part of the body is so vulnerable. This concept precedes all the hangings, garrottings and stranglings of our modern era. 2000 years ago the Roman Emperor Caligula is reported as saying "Oh that the people had but one neck" namely a shared vulnerability so he could slay them all with one stroke. Over the years the neck has appeared in many phrases emphasising its weakness: if you "stick your neck out" you offer your most vulnerable part to your enemy, or if you keep it strong by being "stiff necked" or "brass necked" you are more secure. You "get it in the neck" when you receive punishment or reprimand. If you disappear to some far off "neck of the woods" you make yourself less traceable so reducing your vulnerability. But you can express pride or self confidence with "chin up" and if you treat it gently it can be a source of well-being or pleasure. As Frank Sinatra put it so succinctly to Debbie Reynolds in the Tender Trap "Let's neck". This book, however, is not so concerned with the lethality of blows to the neck as to a whole host of apparently unrelated symptoms, following lesser traumas, which are less identifiable and frequently misdiagnosed. We will consider both together – "neck and neck". My theory is not a 'pain in the neck'.

My Revelation

How did my fascination for the neck arise? After completion of my medical studies and post graduation in 1982 in Moscow, I worked in Delhi for six years and built-up a very successful practice in Integrated Medicine. I combined my medical knowledge and experience with what I had learnt in Traditional and Complementary Medicine. In those days I used conventional or allopathic medicine to treat acute conditions, such as flu, severe migraine, high blood pressure, diarrhoea etc. For treatment of chronic backache, fatigue, IBS, asthma etc, I used acupuncture, herbal remedies (both Ayurveda and Unani), homeopathy, yoga and some massage.

Initially, people were sceptical about this combination of different types of medicine, but as stories and success began to spread, my practice grew. Then, something happened and my attitude towards medicine changed completely – you could almost say a 'EUREKA' moment – when I found the secret of spontaneous and innate healing.

I was invited to Bangkok at short notice to see someone who had mysteriously slipped into a coma. My flight left Delhi at 2AM and I landed just under four hours later. I was totally exhausted. The man who came to meet me wanted me to go directly to the hospital as the patient was in a critical condition. However, I needed a few hours sleep and time to prepare to treat him. He then offered to take me somewhere where I could have quick treatment myself.

I was taken to someone's home near a temple. I was shown into a basement room and asked to lie down. He gently grabbed my neck, but what followed was unbelievably painful. He began to press hard and found some sore spots in the neck, occiput and shoulders. He stretched my neck, twisted it sideways and gave it a sudden jerk to crack my displaced joints. It was a form of manipulation used, I knew, by chiropractors and osteopaths. I then felt a 'gush' of blood into the head and I had a tingling sensation in my brain. The dimly lit room seemed brighter and there wasn't a slightest hint of exhaustion left in my body; I felt instantly 'rejuvenated'. 'What a strange experience!', I thought.

I then went straight to the hospital, feeling fresh, to give the patient some acupuncture.   I also decided to massage his neck and shoulders, as I was convinced that the neck treatment could stimulate the brain – I was already aware of some acupuncture points in the neck which help to combat headaches and dizziness.   However, as he was on a ventilator, it was difficult to stretch and manipulate the area.

As I carried out my treatment, the patient's eyelids flickered and there was some movement in his toes.   I continued to use this therapy, three times a day – it was total guesswork at this point, as I had never used this technique before.   I had also brought some powder of pearl and drops containing musk which are traditional remedies for weakened patients and are known to stimulate the nervous system and increase the chance of revival?   On the third day, success came when the patient opened his eyes and the ventilator was removed. Further treatment followed and the patient recovered.   The doctors believed it was a case of spontaneous recovery, whilst I was totally convinced that the acupressure, neck massage and stimulation of the nervous system did the trick.

Follow up

I then decided to explore further.   I had heard that in a Naturopathy centre in Phillaur, the Punjab, hot water was used to stimulate the neck and spine of most patients once a day.   Hot water was poured down the neck and spine from an aluminium kettle with a long nozzle.   I then went to Jiwan Nagar in Haryana, some four hours drive from Delhi, where I used to hold free medical camps for poor villagers twice a month.

During one of my visits, I was shown a bed with rollers.   The patient lay on the bed, was grabbed by the legs and their neck and upper back were rolled up and down the bed. This treatment was used to massage the neck and shoulder and to stimulate the nerves. Patients with chronic ailments, such as headaches, fatigue, backache, and various nervous disorders were treated with the 'Rolling technique' with some success.   'Why the neck and shoulder?' I wondered.

With my inquisitive and analytical brain ticking, I opened my Anatomy Atlas and began to study the pictures of the neck and back. This showed there were three pairs of neck ganglia (which are a concentration of nerve cells that form nodules) of the sympathetic nervous system. These were said to have a powerful role to play in improving the functions of the various organs in this area and their blood supply. I was not convinced this was the complete answer.

I realised that one pair of the arteries and veins in the neck were hidden away in a canal that runs on either side of the neck vertebrae. This pair of canals is formed by the lateral holes in the wings of the neck vertebrae and by thick sheaths of fibrous tissue. My initial question was: 'why has Nature protected these arteries so well?' No other blood vessels were so treated – except for those in the heart, which beats constantly so the risk of pressure on vital arteries is high. There had to be a reason why they had received such strong protection from the trauma or injury. The logical answer was: these blood vessels must be extremely vital for the very existence of the body.

I began to trace these arteries, which are called Vertebral Arteries, to the brain. I could not believe what I discovered. These arteries supplied blood to the subconscious part of the brain which carries out all the 'automatic 'or 'unconscious' functions of the body. Without this part of the brain, nothing in the body can function. Moreover, it is the most ancient part of the brain in evolution, if we are able to believe in that. Our very existence depends on the blood supplied through these arteries and the waste drained down via the corresponding veins to and from the Subconscious Brain.

The logic is simple. The Conscious Brain appeared later in the evolutionary history, so the arteries that feed it also developed later. Similarly, if cancer develops somewhere in the body, a new network of blood vessels develops to feed it. The blood vessels that developed to feed the Conscious Brain predominantly are known as the Carotid Arteries which are located in the front of the neck and are only protected by muscles; no canals or tubes protect them. They are free-standing.

All vertebrates have Vertebral Arteries, but only mammals, gifted with the Conscious or Cortical Brain, have Carotid Arteries. Nature has made this clear-cut distinction, based upon the type of nervous or mental activities they carry out. At this point, therefore, I must explain the anatomy of the brain.

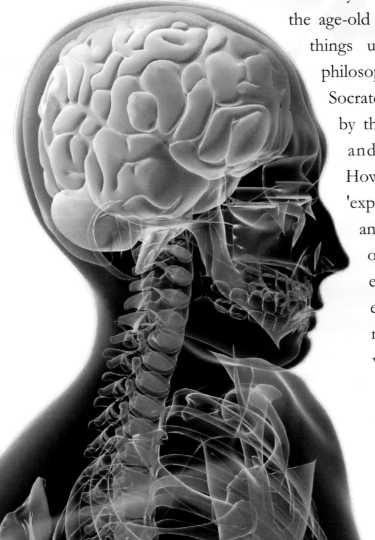

The Brain

The brain is a controversial subject, as the very existence of the subconscious, termed as 'involuntary', 'automatic' or 'unconscious' functions of the brain, is poorly defined or understood by science. Here one has to rely on logic, the age-old method of proving and analyzing things used so brilliantly by the great philosophers such as Aristotle, Plato, and Socrates. Today, the art of logic is replaced by the science of physics, mathematics and chemistry to prove things. However, the Latin word for 'to prove" is 'experiri' to which the words 'experience' and 'experiment' are both related. In other words proof can be by experiment (science), or by experience (logic). It is therefore a mistake to replace one with the other, we still depend heavily on both.

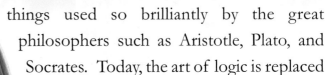

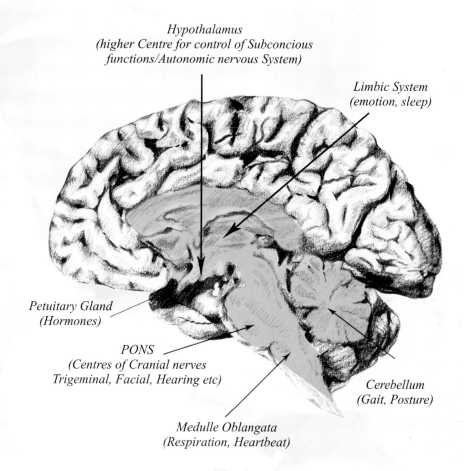

Hypothalamus
(higher Centre for control of Subconcious
functions/Autonomic nervous System)

Limbic System
(emotion, sleep)

Petuitary Gland
(Hormones)

PONS
(Centres of Cranial nerves
Trigeminal, Facial, Hearing etc)

Cerebellum
(Gait, Posture)

Medulle Oblangata
(Respiration, Heartbeat)

Fig. 1

SECTION OF THE BRAIN SHOWING THE SUBCONSCIOUS BRAIN.
THE CONSCIOUS BRAIN IS ABOVE IT.

The Two Brains

The Conscious Brain.

This is known as the Cortical Brain and forms the superficial or outer layers, of the brain. It makes decisions, analyses, makes deductions, uses logic, makes voluntary movements; senses pain, heat, touch, vision, hearing, smell etc.; stores long-term memory, and above all, is responsible for our intellectual function-thinking. The Subconscious Brain or Unconscious Brain deals with everything else. It regulates hormones; maintains body temperature; controls heartbeat, breathing, digestion, appetite, balance, gait, posture, sexual functioning, sleep, energy levels, the immune system, emotions, short-term memory etc. These subconscious functions of the brain are complicated and are beyond our voluntary decisions, or Will, for any effective control. For example, if you walk into a sauna with an extremely high temperature, within seconds of your being there the body's temperature control 'automatically' reacts by raising the heart rate; opening up the pores to secrete sweat; dilating blood vessels etc. The adaptive process cannot be regulated by our conscious brain, which generally works more slowly. If you touch a thorn on a rose stem and, in a quick reflex action, pull your hand away, you do so even before you feel the pain, which is a subconscious reflex action. The Conscious Brain cannot have the capacity to analyze the exact component of food; both the quantity and chemical structure of the ingested matter. The Subconscious Brain does that for us and achieves perfect digestion; the absorption of useful matter and elimination of waste. Thus, Nature made a unique system of control within the body that helps to sustain life and regulate all its functions.

Certain functions of the body are both consciously (voluntarily) and/or unconsciously (involuntarily) controlled. We know breathing is involuntary, taking place at the rate of 16 breaths per minute. Yet, it can be voluntarily controlled. Pearl divers hold their breath for 5 minutes. Yoga and meditation involve breath control. Singing and playing wind instruments require voluntary control of the breath for the desired effect. Similarly, our erect posture can be changed voluntarily. Our skills begin by being a voluntary action but with some practice soon become involuntary, or part of our unconscious. Standing, walking, riding a bicycle, driving, writing, playing a musical instrument all start off by voluntarily exercising certain groups of muscles and then with some training, the control becomes automatic, or involuntary. We do not need to 'use our brain' most of the time. Both speech and writing are perfect examples where thoughts are translated into movement involuntarily or instantly.

One can continue to be alive without the conscious brain, as its role is not entirely vital. Lobotomy, an unfortunate operation performed on psychologically affected people, proves the point. When the frontal lobe of the cortex is removed, the person continues to live normally, except that he or she cannot think, as the intellectual functions no longer exist.

Diseases that affect the Cortical Brain do not affect life processes. Superficial brain haemorrhage, stroke, benign tumours, coma etc. affect the conscious brain and so the heartbeat, breathing and the vital symptoms continue, as these centres are not affected. Somewhere in the world I heard, a man in coma had been kept alive for 22 years with a life-support machine.

A clot travelling through the vertebral arterial network is fatal in a majority of cases. The clot will plug one or the other smaller arteries cutting off the blood supply to vital centres of the brain. Thus, the vertebral arteries feeding the subconscious brain are vital to the person's survival.

In a very crude way, we can see the effect of Halal or Kosher methods of slaughtering animals. When the carotid arteries of the neck are severed by this method, the conscious brain dies but, because the vertebral arteries are not severed, the subconscious brain continues to function for a few minutes. The heart beats and so the circulation of blood continues. This helps to flush out blood from the flesh as the bleeding through the severed (cut) carotid arteries continues. The meat is 'freed' from toxins in the blood and is supposedly tastier than the flesh of animals killed instantly. I must stress I intend no disrespect to the practitioners by using this as an example.

Just as the lungs and heart are protected by the ribcage, the brain, which is the most important and delicate organ of the body, is protected by a tough skull. There are also tough membranes that lie beneath the skull. Finally, there is fluid that bathes the outer and inner surface of the brain. In fact, the brain is buoyant in this fluid so, if the head moves, the brain (like a buoy), remains relatively static and its surface does not collide with the skull. The brain is kept safe, while its owner is jumping, running, skipping etc, by this fluid, known as Cerebro Spinal Fluid or CSF.

The Subconscious Brain lies beneath the thick layer of the Cortical or Conscious Brain. Thus, in an accident when the outer surface is shaken-up, one suffers concussion and looses consciousness. The heart and lungs, whose control centres are located deep in the subconscious brain, often remain unaffected and continue to function. If you imagine a cauliflower or broccoli, the outer flower is the cortical, or conscious brain and the stalks, or stems, in the centre represent the subconscious brain. These stalks are tougher; more resilient and are also protected by the flower on top. (stalks have fibres which are tough).

The Subconscious Brain.

I do not intend to go into the detailed anatomy of the Subconscious Brain but some description is necessary to explain where things are located. If you look at the brain in a standing position, it is like a five storey building. On the top floor lies the Cerebrum, the Cortical or Conscious Brain, with the higher centres of intellect: logic, voluntary movements, analysis of pain, light, sound, colour, decision making etc. The fourth floor (Diencaphalon) consists of a split level flat. The upper portion (Thalamus) houses all the nerve fibres, or cables, going to and from the Cortical Brain. The lower portion, called the Hypothalamus, which is below the Thalamus, houses the headquarters of the Subconscious Brain. This is the command centre, from where instructions are given to all the automatic or involuntary functions of the body. This is also the intelligence centre, which receives and analyses the goings-on in the body. The passage of food through the intestines; heart rate; breathing; the emotional state of the body; hormone levels etc, are all controlled from here. The Hypothalamus is also the appetite centre; the thermostat or body temperature regulator; circulation centre; water retention centre; short-term memory; sexual urge (libido and orgasm); emotional controls; labour; milk production; stomach acid secretion; adaptation to sun, altitude or extreme weather conditions. Along with numerous other automatic functions these are all controlled from this most important centre of the Subconscious Brain.

The Hypothalamus has a rear chamber filled with brain fluid (CSF). Its roof has the analytical centres of emotions - rage, passion, fear, sorrow, jealousy, revenge: we feel them here and react through the Hypothalamus which expresses emotions via hormones.   At the rear end of this chamber, we have the Pineal Gland which produces the hormone Melatonin, the night hormone responsible for rest and sleep.

Just below the Hypothalamus, and in front of it lies the highly protected Pituitary Gland. This gland rests in a chamber guarded on three sides by a part of the skull called the Saddle. This is where all the hormones are regulated and is the true headquarters of our hormonal system such as the thyroid, adrenals, ovaries, testes, melanin production (for pigmentation of the skin). The Hypothalamus and Pituitary work together as the former gives the commands which the latter executes. Our immune system; sense of wellbeing; energy; healing power; stress levels; ageing are all controlled by these two interlinked structures of the Subconscious Brain.

The third floor houses the Mid Brain (Mesencephalon). This part of the brain maintains consciousness, so keeps us awake and alert. Chronic fatigue and excessive sleep – like Narcolepsy – are related to this part of the brain. This part also analyses our hearing and vision.

The second level of the brain consists of the Pons (meaning 'bridge'). This is the link that connects the Midbrain with the Brain Stem and Cerebellum, which is the mini brain, lying beneath the main brain. The surfaces of these two 'brains' look similar but have completely different functions.   The Cerebellum controls posture and fine tuning of gait; writing; acquired skills like playing a musical instrument, dancing, knitting and all the activities we do automatically without being seriously 'mindful'. Some scientists think it is the most intelligent part of the brain .It communicates with Nature and adapts to its changes.

The Pons has the nuclei, or nerve centres, for the eye muscles, inner ear, facial muscles etc. Here also lies the centre that controls the rythmicity of breathing. If something is not right here, the result is palpitations.

The lowest part of the brain consists of the stem of the brain called the Medulla Oblongata, as it is oblong–shaped. This connects the brain with the spinal cord that runs down the entire length of the back. The most important centre in this part is the one that controls both breathing and heartbeat. The forces with which these vital organs function are automatically controlled from these two centres. There are many nerve centres here that control facial expression, tongue movement, gum sensations, teeth, face, taste buds, hearing etc. Thus the Medulla Oblongata is also a very important part of the brain. Moreover, all the information passing to the various parts of the brain from the entire body and vice versa, pass through the nerve fibres located here.

I cannot stress enough the importance of the Subconscious Brain. As I go along, I will explain how disease and wellbeing are linked to this part of the brain in the vast majority of cases and in particular the influence on it of the neck.

The Discovery

When the apple fell on my head, I discovered that the subconscious brain has its own circulatory network, quite independently, except that, at a higher level of the brain, it is re-enforced by a branch of the carotid arteries, namely the internal carotid artery, as a back-up. This enforcement happens so that additional blood can be supplied to the Pituitary Gland, to produce vital hormones, to the Hypothalamus, or Headquarters of the Subconscious Brain and to the other important centres.

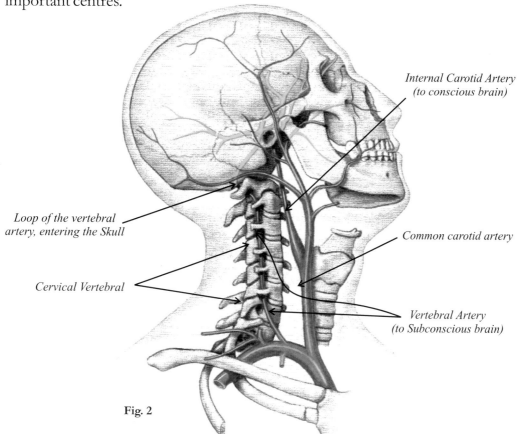

Internal Carotid Artery
(to conscious brain)

Loop of the vertebral
artery, entering the Skull

Common carotid artery

Cervical Vertebral

Vertebral Artery
(to Subconscious brain)

Fig. 2

Branches of Arteries emerging from the Heart.

I began to study the anatomy of the neck. It has seven flat bodied vertebrae, in a span of some 15 cm, whereas the entire back, which is normally over half a metre long, has only 17 vertebrae. These flat vertebrae of the neck are light and flexible. Our sensory organs, such as our eyes, ears and nose are directional so our head has to turn frequently to see, hear and smell. The rest of the spine is less flexible. Here lies the problem. Since the neck is flexible, it is more prone to traumas and dislocation. Thus in terms of pain or stiffness, our neck gives us more trouble than any other part of the body.

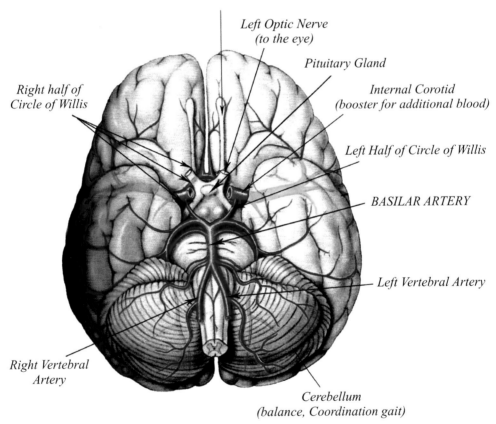

(OLFACTORY BULB FOR SMELL)

Left Optic Nerve
(to the eye)

Pituitary Gland

Right half of
Circle of Willis

Internal Corotid
(booster for additional blood)

Left Half of Circle of Willis

BASILAR ARTERY

Left Vertebral Artery

Right Vertebral
Artery

Cerebellum
(balance, Coordination gait)

Fig. 3

Blood Vessels (Arteries) on the inferior Surface of the brain

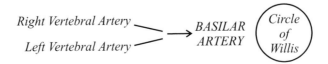

Right Vertebral Artery → BASILAR ARTERY Circle of Willis

Left Vertebral Artery

The vertebrae of the neck move very freely in the top section so that the rotation of the head is possible. This is facilitated by the two vertebrae at the top, called the Atlas and Axis. The second vertebra, the Axis, has a finger-like projection around which the first one, the Atlas, rotates. The head rests on the Atlas. The lower five vertebrae of the neck move to facilitate the rotation of the head, but do not do so as freely as the Atlas.

As I mentioned earlier, the vertebral arteries, our better 'life source', run through a pair of canals located in the first five vertebrae of the neck, inside their wings (see photo of cervical vertebrae in front of the book Fig. A). Then they emerge; make a loop and join together to form the Basiler Artery at the base of the brain, which is located on the lower surface of the Medulla Oblongata. At this point, it is already inside the skull, so its protection is ensured. Here Nature has a shortcoming in that it has protected the vital Vertebral Arteries except for 2cms or so, (Fig. A) when they come out of the canals and form the loop before entering the protected space of the skull. Thus, between the base of the Axis and the occiput (lower skull), the arteries are covered not by bones but by a sheath of thick ligament. Unfortunately, ligaments are not bones and after head injuries, whiplash injuries, falls, traumas of labour etc., these can tear or get pulled. This results in the compression of the arteries, despite their strength and elasticity, whenever the neck muscles get stiff from stress, excessive computer use etc.

Many head and neck injuries caused by trauma result in dislocation of the facet joints of the cervical vertebrae. In my opinion, the most common are of the first four vertebrae. The dislocation causes misalignment of the cervical spine. The shifted vertebrae pull or twist the vertebral arteries. The blood flow through the Vertebral Arteries is then restricted or the flow becomes turbulent. This compression of the arteries ultimately causes a malfunction of the Subconscious Brain, often with disastrous consequences.

Effect on the Brain

The brain cells are highly specialized and they need 'fuel' to function all the time. They do not have any reserve fat or carbohydrate storage facility. They instantly utilize what is available. Moreover, there exists a strict blood-brain barrier: not everything that is carried by blood can permeate into brain cells. This barrier facilitates the passage of safe products and chemicals to the brain, again ensuring that there is no damage done to the brain cells. Oxygen and glucose are easily accessible to the brain cells. In fact, the brain cells are highly susceptible to a decrease in the supply of oxygen and glucose levels. We know very well that when sugar levels in the blood, or the brain drop, the effect is hypoglycaemia (hypo- less, glycogen, or sugar) and is alarming, as the person experiences shivering, fainting sensation, a cold sweat, panic etc. Lack of oxygen (as at high altitude) causes palpitations, tingling, an irregular breathing pattern, fainting etc.

Alcohol, narcotic drugs, tranquillizers, tobacco, sedatives, certain chemotherapy drugs etc., cross the blood-brain barrier and reach the brain cells to produce their respective effect. Some drugs, especially those used recreationally such as Speed, Ecstasy etc., are chemically engineered to break this barrier. Alcohol's effect on the brain is traditionally so obvious. First, it relaxes the mind, and then excites it, before the drinker collapses into a comatose state.

The oxygen and glucose supply to the brain are together the key controller of its function. We all know that if the oxygen supply to the brain is stopped for approximately four minutes, the brain cells change and can die. That is how sensitive they are. Other cells, like muscles and bone scan survive for several hours, or days. If the blood supply to the toes is blocked, by diabetic or frostbite conditions, the necrosis, or death of the cells, takes a while to develop. With my special massage, I have helped several patients with slight necrosis (black tissue in the toes) to regain their functions and to regenerate the tissues again. After a snake bite, it is common practice to tie the arm, or thigh, very tightly with a rope so that the blood supply is totally cut-off, until help is received. This may take several hours and after anti-venom treatment is given, the compressed limb recovers its full function.

In suicide by hanging, death comes quickly. As the blood-flow to the brain is cut-off, as the breathing is obstructed, the person goes to sleep and doesn't feel anything. Just before death, there is a sudden jerk and all voluntary and involuntary functions cease. At the very last minute, the person may involuntarily urinate or defecate as the corresponding sphincters dilate.

These are dramatic situations. In the majority of cases, it is the malfunctioning of the brain tissue and the various centres of the Sub-conscious Brain which matters most. In my experience and with logical (non-scientific) analysis, I have found that if the blood flow to the Subconscious Brain is reduced by say 40%, it begins to malfunction and chronic fatigue sets in. The person feels tired, lethargic, listless etc. and most voluntary functions, such as walking, talking, thinking, making decisions, comprehension etc., slow down as well. The nerve fibres from the Conscious Brain pass through the Subconscious Brain. The centres for gait, emotions etc., are located here, so their functions are also affected.

If the blood flow is reduced further, by about say 60%, the person experiences headaches, nausea, sickness, extreme fatigue, loss of muscle power, extreme sensitivity to light, dizziness, imbalance etc. If the blood flow to the Subconscious Brain is reduced by more that say 80%, then the person gets panic attacks, vertigo, epileptic fits, acute tinnitus, sees flashing lights, palpitations and has tremors in the body etc. If the blood to the Subconscious Brain is reduced by more than 80%, then fainting occurs and a person will collapse. All parts of the body shut-down and only the heart and lungs are kept active, because Nature tries to conserve oxygen for the functioning of these two vital organs. If, however, the oxygen supply through blood stops for 4 minutes, the brain then suffers irreversible changes. Its proteins change and the cell walls loose their functions. If, on the other hand, the body is in a frozen state and the heart stops because of that, such as drowning in an ice-cold lake, then the cells of the heart and respiration centres are kept inert. The brain tissue in this state does not go through irreversible changes. This feature can be used in heart surgery. While I was a student in Moscow, we observed how open-heart surgery was performed by cooling the blood to 4 degreesC. The requirement for oxygen in the brain decreases to a minimum in freezing conditions. Animals, such as bears, can hibernate for months during the cold winter months.

In the early 70's, a strange experiment was carried out by international scientists in Delhi. An expert of Yoga, known as a Yogi, was buried alive in a coffin and his heart was monitored by an ECG machine. His heart slowed down to about 10 beats per minute; enough to supply the basic amount of oxygen to the brain. He was in a hibernative state. He remained there for almost 7 days. When dug out, he was able to breathe and function normally. This yogi used his powers of the Conscious Brain and suppressed, or slowed down the heart beat, a function normally reserved for the Subconscious Brain.

Decreased blood supply to the brain can diminish its functions. If there is anaemia or low blood pressure, the effect is obvious. The person feels very tired, has mild palpitations, yawns and sighs a lot, feels dizziness, has headaches and has a 'sinking feeling' in the heart. Again, after a heavy meal, the blood rushes to the stomach and intestines to aid digestion by churning the stomach to break-up food, increase gastric juice secretion, provide for movement of food through the intestines and absorption of digested food etc. This deprives the brain of blood and so one feels very sleepy and often edgy if one has to work. This is why, in many countries, people take an afternoon siesta in order to avoid being underactive after lunch.

Before menstruation, blood rushes to the lower abdomen to form a reserve in the pelvic region, in preparation for a sudden haemorrhage. This draws blood away from the brain, resulting in a range of physical and psychological symptoms known as Pre-menstrual Syndrome. About 3-7 days before the onset of the period, women may feel agitated, exhausted, emotional (often unreasonably), panicky, restless, suffer sleeplessness etc. Water retention and painful breasts are hormone- related and they are caused by functions of the Pituitary Gland which controls and regulates hormones.

The Role of CSF

Earlier, I mentioned Cerebro Spinal Fluid (CSF) in which the brain 'floats'. This fluid penetrates various chambers and canal ways, located deep inside the brain. These are the backwaters of the sea of CSF which cover the outer surface of the brain. They are called ventricles. This fluid contains some oxygen, the level of which is the same as can be absorbed by water. However, the level of glucose in the CSF is substantial, so it can be an additional supply of fuel for both the inner and outer surfaces of the brain. It also contains some minerals which are dissolved in the liquid. The CSF cannot diffuse deep into the brain, so it is a secondary, but important, source of fuel for the brain.

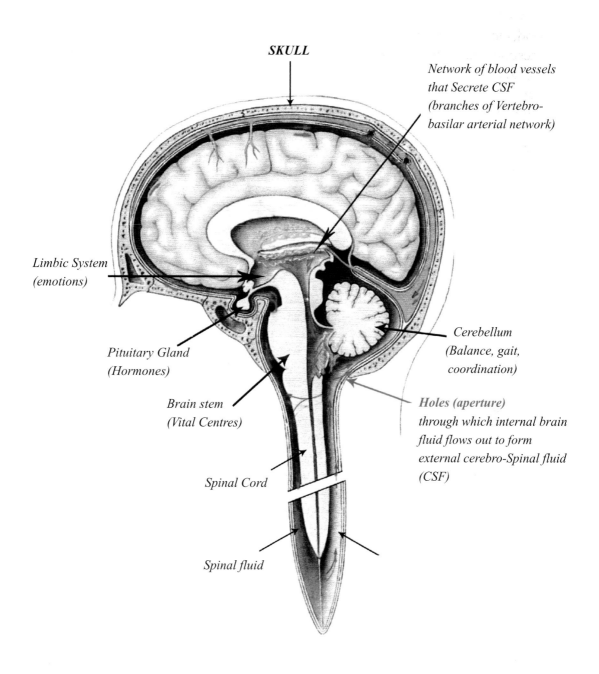

Fig. 4

FORMATION and CIRCULATION of Cerebro - Spinal Fluid (CSF) or Brain Fluid

If there is a leakage of this fluid after an epidural injection – in the case of anaesthesia for painless labour or pelvic surgery – the patient will suffer headaches, extreme fatigue and dizziness.

If excess fluid accumulates as in hydrocephaly (a large head, swollen with fluid) in babies, the brain surfaces are squashed due to the hydraulic pressure and the result is poor development of mental and physical capabilities and the child is often retarded.

Blood flow to the brain is more vital than CSF circulation because of the former's oxygen supplying capabilities, through its Red Blood Cells. Cranial Osteopaths generally help to improve the CSF circulation to the brain by gentle manipulation. My technique, which I call the 'Ali Technique', helps to improve both the blood and the CSF to the brain. The results from this technique are more prominent and long-lasting.

Restriction of Blood Supply

In order to understand how important constant and ample supply of blood to the brain is, we must look at the negative side. This is a purely logical approach. What happens to the body and its functioning when there is a reduced supply of blood to the brain? If you look at the extreme case of a stroke, when a blood clot forms in the heart due to an irregular heart beat, it travels along an artery and plugs one of the smaller blood vessels, the corresponding area of the brain is instantly starved of oxygen and glucose. That part of the brain soon dies. If the clot travels through the carotid artery to the cortical, or conscious brain, there will be instant loss of muscle power on one side of the body and the person may even become unconscious. If the clot travels to the left half of the brain, where the speech centre is located in a right-handed person, there is a loss of speech. For that to happen to a left-handed person, the clot must travel to the right side of the brain. This is so because the nerve fibres from the brain cells cross over in the brain stem area to connect to the opposite side of the body.

If the clot travels up the Vertebral Arteries, the Subconscious Brain is starved of oxygen instantly. Depending on where the clot gets stuck, the corresponding part of the brain dies. If blood flow to the brain stem is blocked, then there is instant death, as both the heart and respiratory centres of the brain stop functioning. A clot along the Vertebral Artery is usually fatal, which is again a proof that the Subconscious Brain is vital to our existence and the arteries that feed it are the most important blood vessels, besides the coronary(or heart) arteries, in the entire body.

A clot plugs an artery like dirt in a drain pipe and it cuts off the blood flow beyond it. As I said, this is an extreme situation, but in the vast majority of cases, there is only a reduction in blood supply. Unless a tumour compresses one or other branch of the said arteries, the main obstruction takes place either in the section of the arteries inside the vertebral canal, or in a loop section of these blood vessels.

Causes
The following are some of the causes of narrowing of the canal in the neck, gathered by me over 20 years of practice:

1. **Misalignment of the neck vertebrae** due to whiplash injuries, forceps or Ventouse delivery; head and neck injuries; boxing; tumbling, as in a skiing accident; falls from heights or horseback; walking into glass doors; hitting the head on a beam when walking; excessive dental work; long anaesthesia during surgery (when the head is pushed back and there is no resistance); cutting the jaw; breaking the nose; an embryo lying with the face squashed in the uterus especially with twins; being dropped as a child or falling from a cot; tumbling downstairs; motor cycle accidents; brawls or domestic violence; habitually sleeping on the stomach for many years; lying with the head twisted in rubble after an earthquake; frequent bungee jumping etc.

2. **Compression of the discs** of the vertebrae of the neck, resulting in narrowing or kinks, in the vertebral arteries. Causes include doing frequent yogic headstands without preparation; objects falling on the head; head-on collisions in Rugby; hitting the head on taxi or car doors; falling head down; diving into the wall of a swimming pool; very rapid labour through a tight birth canal ('Champagne cork' birth within 30 minutes to 1 hour); severe contraction during labour with the opening of the birth canal tightly closed, labour in the breech position with strong contraction on the head of the baby; motor car accident, when it overturns and lies upside down; a tree falling on the head; earthquake with trauma to the head when the ceiling collapses; rod or stick hitting in fights; accident of stuntmen when objects hit the head; a rod falling on the head whilst weight-lifting, etc.

3. **Sudden lateral movement of the head and neck** due to falling-off a horse; skiing accidents; football injuries, punches on the cheeks as in boxing or fights; martial arts injuries to the side of the face from kicking sideways; car being hit from the side; spinning in a car accident; facial surgeries under anaesthesia; difficult extraction of molar, or premolar tooth (on the side of the mouth), etc.

4. **Repetitive movements of the head and neck** as in dancing; frequent use of the telephone with the head tilted to one side; sports injuries (Rugby, American football), etc. The vertebral artery circulation is also affected by a very stiff neck.

5. **Poor mobility as a result of calcium deposits** on the facet joints of the cervical vertebrae; working posture; narrowing of the spinal canal (where the spinal cord is located) due to disc protruding in the spinal canal causing pain and stiffness of the neck; crushing of the neck vertebrae from old fractures etc.

6. **Neck stiffness due to poor mobility** caused by excessive computer use (typically more than 6 hours a day), driving, knitting, sedentary desk jobs, playing the violin with the neck held in the same position for a long time, lying in bed for many days (typically due to fractures of the spinal bones), using neck collars for many days, etc. Arab men who wear head gears (not turbans) have to fix their head up right as the wooden square frame they wear is likely to slip. They are very conscious of that embarrassing situation. Strong wind awkward movements, running, bending down can make the head gear slip. They have a lot of neck pain.

7. **Neck stiffness due to imposed conditions** such as Osteoporosis, when the neck shrinks; Ankylosis, or fusion of the joints of the cervical spine due to an auto-immune disease; putting titanium discs in the spine; fixing a rod (Harrington's) in the neck to immobilize it in extreme neck damage or degenerative scoliosis, arthritis of the joints of the neck; paraplegia (paralysis from the neck down after a spinal injury) etc.

8. **If plaque (atherosclerosis) is formed** in the inner lining of vertebral arteries due to high cholesterol, smoking, diabetes. The reduction of blood flow is permanent. People have frequent "Mini" strokes, (TIA), faint, vertigo, tinnitus as in old age.

These conditions severely affect the neck, whose shape and functioning are modified. Blood flow to the brain is then simultaneously reduced.

There are other causes which affect the general blood circulation and deprive the brain. These may be temporary or long-term. After a heavy meal the blood forms a depot around the stomach area. This reduces the total amount of blood reaching the brain. Thus, one feels drowsy or lethargic after a meal. Before menstruation begins there is a tendency to pelvic congestion. The blood forms a depot around the uterus, in case there is a severe haemorrhaging during the period. Acute blood-loss due to blood-letting, trauma or surgery, blood donation, severe dehydration, leeching, anaemia, very low blood pressure, arrhythmic heartbeat (missing beats), atrial fibrillation- when the heart 'flutters' etc., all reduce the amount of oxygen to the brain. Those teenagers who grow very quickly, which is quite a common phenomenon nowadays, can have very long necks. If they also suffer from low blood pressure the brain will get less blood and it will function poorly. Such teenagers are often tired and irritable, suffering from lack of concentration, poor immune system, excessive acne, cravings for sweets or chocolates, insomnia etc. In aerobatics, negative G-force can cause blackout for a brief period. They see pink when they have positive G-force (the opposite) while flying.

Imagine you are watering the garden. Some areas get more water than others. That depends on the uneven surface density of the grass, distance from the source etc. If the pressure of the water in the hose pipe is low and not enough flows through it, those areas will receive very little water; some areas will only receive a trickle. Similar things happen in the brain. There are numerous blood vessels and they are not perfect in shape and size (rather like our face, eyes nose, thumb prints etc.). Even when the pressure, or volume, of blood running through it is adequate, the various parts of the brain get varying amounts of blood.

The Carotid Arteries run almost unobstructed and the chances of their compression are small except when plaque is formed due to excess cholesterol in blood. That is not the same with the Vertebral Arteries. There are too many variables, especially as most of the tunnels through which they travel consist of movable cervical vertebrae. They can shift sideways or forward and backwards. Then, in the upper part, they are covered by the roof that is made of sheaths of fibrous tissue which can tear or flatten when pulled by the highly mobile first vertebra of the spine.

The chances of obstruction to the smooth flow of blood through this pair of arteries are very high. This is the price we homosapiens have to face for walking erect. Our predecessors, the four-legged animals, moved horizontally and so the blood from the heart went straight through the canals to the brain. The pressure was adequate to overcome any mild compression or minor kinks. However, when a dog sits too long on its hind legs begging it sometimes goes to sleep and falls over. Humans face the same problem by walking vertically. We have to pump blood against gravity so even the slightest resistance along the path of the canals can result in poor irrigation of the brain. Giraffes, when swinging their head, are often disorientated (they probably feel dizzy) because of their long neck. Reaching for green leaves on the top of the tree has been made easy, but eating grass and then moving the head up can cause discomfort.

The key issue is that different parts of the Subconscious Brain have different functions. The symptoms that arise from malfunction of various nerve or control centres, or of major functions of the body can vary. Some may be psychological in nature, while others could be physical (palpitation, extreme fatigue, headaches, imbalance etc.) but the cause is the same: reduced blood supply.

These symptoms will be discussed in the next chapter under the heading 'The Ali Syndrome', which is how it became known in my clinic.

Stress

We conclude this chapter by talking about the role stress plays in increasing the demand of oxygen in the brain and simultaneously cutting-off the supply chain. It is a bizarre reaction. In stress, it is obvious that the brain cells will be hyperactive and so they need more blood. This high demand brings in more fluid to the brain (CSF) because it too has glucose and some oxygen. As the fluid accumulates in the brain canals, cisterns and the skull, the pressure on the brain surface increases. This tightens the neck very quickly to stop more fluid formation. This tightening of the neck muscles causes reduction of blood flow through vertebral arteries. The subconscious brain then gets less blood.

In Meningitis, there is increased fluid pressure in the brain and thus the first symptom is tightness of the neck muscles. The Dutch name for Meningitis is 'Nek Kramp' (neck cramp). When a child cries, the neck becomes very tight with stress. Barking dogs are stressed and their neck muscles also tighten-up.

There is a short-term or acute stress, like a burst of anger. When the situation calms down the neck muscles relax. Chronic conditions, however, stress the body and tighten the neck permanently in anticipation. This is the Conditional Reflex, as described in Pavlovian experiments with dogs where flashing lights caused stomach secretion, even when food was not actually given.

Stress, therefore, can cause prolonged reduction of blood flow to the subconscious brain. That, in my opinion, is the logical explanation of why stress is linked to so many diseases. The failure of a particular brain centre leads to the breaking down of functions of the corresponding organs or systems.

I have not found any mention in Medicine where scientists have been able to explain why prolonged stress causes us so much harm. I sincerely hope that sceptics will accept my hypothesis and carry out experiments to prove or disprove it.

The Ali Syndrome

First of all, what is a syndrome? One could say a causeless condition.

A disease is characterised by the presence of a cause. Thus, bronchitis, viral meningitis, arthritis, cystitis etc., are called diseases. We can pin point the cause like inflammation (a suffix 'itis' means inflammation), a virus, bacteria etc.

A syndrome is not a disease as it is difficult to point out the 'cause' of this condition. In reality, a Syndrome is a collection of symptoms which may, or may not, be linked. There is usually no single cause that manifests as symptoms. Here are some examples:

1. **Down's Syndrome**

   The cause is an extra 21st pair of chromosomes. There are three instead of two prints of the chromosome. The syndrome is characterised by 'mongoloid' (slit eyes, round face) face, mental retardation, and defects in the cardiovascular system.

2. **Polycystic Ovarian Syndrome (PCOS)**

   This is characterised by multiple cysts in the ovary. This syndrome comprises dysfunction of periods, weight gain, facial hair, insulin-resistance (which could lead to diabetes) and acne.

3. **Irritable Bowel Syndrome (IBS)**

   This is characterised by frequent diarrhoea, bloating, abdominal cramps, occasional constipation, indigestion, flatulence etc. The actual cause of such varying symptoms is not known, but they are often present in a batch.

The Ali Syndrome

The Ali Syndrome is not a disease, even though we know it results from poor blood supply to the Subconscious Brain, from whatever cause. The symptoms vary in intensity and may appear in various permutations and combinations according to the area of the Subconscious Brain most affected. These include the Limbic system, the Pineal Gland, and the Hypothalamus-Pituitary which work in a partnership. I will discuss the symptoms according to each such location.

The Limbic System

(Limbus – border, between the conscious and subconscious brain). Symptoms include:

a) Loss of drives: loss of libido, desire to do things and motivation.

b) Loss of short-term memory, also storage and retrieval of memory.

c) Loss of smell.

d) Difficulty in chewing, licking and swallowing.

e) Emotional disturbances, such as mood swings, depression, panic attacks, anxiety, becoming angry over small trivial things.

The Pineal Gland

This gland, located at the rear-end of the Hypothalamus area, secretes Melatonin, a hormone which is only produced at night. It is the main regulator of sleep. If cortisol (adrenaline) helps you to carry-out your daytime activities, such as working, digestion, even just staying awake, then melatonin helps you in rest and repose. The repair work of the wear and tear of the body, synthesis of blood cells, healing of cuts, bruises, traumas, replenishing the body's energy, removal of waste from the tissues, helping the liver to replenish energy are all carried out at night when the body is asleep. Thus, Melatonin is as vital as Cortisol, the main daytime hormone.

The blood vessels that feed the Pineal Gland also carry Melatonin secretion to the rest of the body. Malfunction, caused primarily by the failure of the vertebra basilar arterial network, can therefore have serious consequences. First of all, the Day-Night Circadian cycle is reversed. You are awake and 'buzzing' with thoughts at night and very tired and lethargic during the day. In other words, you have permanent Jet-lag. Medicine has called it insomnia, but if you look at it carefully, it is the alteration of the day and night cycle. True Insomnia, or lack of sleep, is when you don't sleep at all; day or night.

Some years ago, it was very fashionable to take synthetic Melatonin. It was thought to be a wonder drug. Some even took it for "rejuvenation" of the body. It may have helped some people to get slightly better sleep, but it didn't do much else. The message from the retina of the eye confirms that it's dark outside and the Pineal Gland begins to secrete Melatonin. The repair and replenishing of the body's energy is flagged up. If someone puts the light on in the room, the Melatonin production and secretion stops instantly. The person is then wide awake and finds himself in difficulty, as going back to sleep will take some time. Thus light, or darkness, determines its function.

Melatonin also helps the maturation of sperm and eggs; a function which is very delicate and requires a lot of energy. The energy depot in the microscopic sperm cells is so phenomenal that they can swim with great speed, in relation to their size, for up to five days. What a power cell it is! It then head-buts its way through the tough wall, or membrane, of the egg cell to fertilize it. That energy is almost celestial. Sperm and egg production and release is a night time activity.

Men get an erection in the early hours of the morning due to the sperm maturation by the production of Testosterone in the Testes. Women ovulate at night, as is seen in the sudden rise in body temperature in the early hours of the morning. Before the new ovulation-detection kit was discovered, it was the body temperature that was recorded to identify the 'peak', which signified ovulation day.

Thus, sleep is essential for reproductive functions. I am quite sure that natural sleep is better than that induced by drugs.

Hypothalamus and Pituitary

The Hypothalamus instructs the Pituitary to secrete specific hormones. Thus, they work together where the Hypothalamus analyses the situation in the body or mind and then commands the Pituitary to secrete the right, or predicted, amount of the given hormone.

This is the most important partnership in the entire body. The Hypothalamus analyses information (through the nerves) coming from the brain, the organs, the skin, blood vessels etc and then sends a corresponding message for the release of the right type and quantity of hormones. The hormone is released into the blood directly and within seconds, transported to all target receptors for quick action. If the Hypothalamus were to target many organs at the same time, through the nerves, it would be spending a lot of time and energy.

For example, if you are in a stressful situation and you need to react immediately, here is how the chain reaction starts: the eyes send a message to the brain which instructs the Hypothalamus to respond. It analyses the information and makes an instantaneous decision for a response strategy. It commands the Pituitary to stimulate the adrenal glands (located above the kidneys) with a stimulating hormone called ACTH. The adrenal glands then secrete Adrenaline, or Cortisol, which is transported via blood to the heart, lungs, muscles, sweat glands etc. The heart beats faster, the breathing rate increases, muscles tighten, the metabolic rate in muscles increases to produce more energy, sweating increases to 'cool' the body etc. Nature has created hormones to do multi-tasking with minimum loss of time and energy.

The Hypothalamus is thus the main 'Intelligence' of the body. The soul, or life force, or the representation of the creator in us, is located in the Hypothalamus. In the universe, or Nature too, there must be a 'Hypothalamus' which controls the solar system, the weather, seasons, climate change as a response to human activities on earth. We simply do not know who, or what, is controlling this harmony. Our body is just a part of that universal system. I am grateful to that Universal Creator that I have been gifted to understand a tiny part of that amazing force that is controlling everything that is happening within us. The interesting thing is that we can exercise some control over that autonomic world with some training of the conscious brain. I have walked over hot marble in the Taj Mahal at midday; held my breath for 1 minute 12 seconds; turned my hand hot or cold at will; elongated my fingers by over a centimetre at will; slowed down my heart rate by 20%, slept without a blanket at a temperature of below 10 degrees C. I am not boasting, but meditation and breath control, over a period of a number of years, can help anyone do this. There are people who have gone even further. I know of a person who did 'Samadhi', a higher yogic method of stopping heart and breathing activity altogether to slip into a hibernation and finally death. It's hard to believe this, but it does happen in India and in Buddhist practices.

There are numerous caves in Tibet where mummified bodies of such monks are still to be found. In Gui, in the Spiti Valley, where I often trek, there is one such mummified monk in a small temple. The mummy is over 500 years old and is totally intact. No one, however, has done any internal examination. There are several caves in the Tabo villages where Buddhist Monks went in Samadhi after completion of their worldly mission in their current life .They sat in the Lotus position, controlled breath, heart rate, cut off from feeling the environment, remained in trance and stepped into Samadhi. Call it euthanasia or a spiritual journey, it's your choice.

The main parameters of the life force, the immune system, adaptation and homeostasis, are entirely controlled and managed by the Hypothalamus-Pituitary complex as follows:

1. The Immune System

This protects us from harm by neutralizing, or destroying, invading bodies. If this is a living bacterium, or virus, the body's immune system produces antibodies to neutralize it. Since viruses thrive inside our cells, hiding from the lymphocytes (the immigration officers, or detectors, of our body) in the blood, the antibodies or interferon are secreted with some difficulty. These particles either attack the viruses directly or attack the cells that carry the viruses. Against fungi, however, there is very little defence. They have a spore, or protective cover, which is hard to penetrate or analyse the chemical formula to then match with a defensive antibody or particles, that would contain their growth or activity.

If the particles are non-living: pollen, seeds or nuts, pollutants, gluten in wheat, egg protein, dog or cat hair, etc., the body's reaction is through the allergy response.   The Hypothalamus identifies these allergens after receiving information from lymphocytes (white blood cells in the blood) and initiates a chemical-hormonal response to the situation. The hormone released by the Basophils (another type of white blood cells) is Histamine. This hormone tries to eliminate the invading allergens by increasing mucous secretion in the body. This causes a runny nose, sneezing, watery and itchy eyes, swollen eyes, clogged nose, a blocked bronchial tract, which can bring on an asthma attack.

Sometimes the body tries to throw off the allergen (non-living particles) through the skin and so one gets eczema, hives, rashes etc. In extreme circumstances, when the body is highly sensitized, as in a nut or shellfish allergy, it tries to stop the entry of these products by massive swelling of the eyes, lips, throat, bronchioles etc, and the breathing stops. This is called Anaphylactic shock. Such patients carry injections containing powerful anti- histamines, or immunosuppressants, that stop the body's over-the-top reaction, which can have fatal consequences.

By the way, an allergic reaction produced by histamines in the body is a good thing. That is to say that the Immune System is functioning well, but unfortunately, the actual reaction can be very unpleasant. Runny nose, sneezing, asthma, itchy eyes and skin, unpleasant-looking rashes on the body etc, are major irritants. We take anti-histamines to block the histamine so that it cannot produce such annoying symptoms. In an ideal world we should use natural methods of desensitization so that the body does not respond so violently and becomes more tolerant.

Sometimes the body's own tissues, like joint surfaces, skin, eyes, gut, kidneys etc, become the target for the immune system. Due to some unexplained condition, some cells or protein structures in the above mentioned tissue go through irreversible changes. The cells, or proteins, become 'foreign' or an allergen to the body's detective cells: lymphocytes. The Hypothalamus receives a message saying that some traitors have 'changed their loyalty to the body'. The angry immune system goes out in full force to destroy these cells, causing a very undesirable reaction called 'Autoimmune Disease'. The body tries to destroy its own tissue because of some misinterpretation. These diseases are Rheumatoid Arthritis, Lupus, Psoriasis, Vitiligo (white patches), Crohn's Disease, Ulcerative Collitis, Nephritis (kidney disease) Scleroderma (when the skin hardens and acquires a leather-like texture), Hashimoto's Thyroid Disease etc.

These conditions are difficult to treat as we still do not know why these tissues become denatured. The Hypothalamus, or the immune system, is doing its job well, even though serious suffering may result. Steroids and strong immunosuppressants are used to symptomatically treat these conditions. I have some solutions to this problem and they will be discussed later.

The Immune System is an extended function of the Innate Healing Power. Its main role is to protect us from foreign bodies, or particles, from settling down in the body. Imagine the opposite, as in the case of AIDS (Acquired Immuno Deficiency Syndrome), where the Immune System functions poorly. All sorts of viral, bacterial and fungal infections (for example from using too many antibiotics for bacterial infections) slowly destroy the body. It results in death.

The Pituitary-Hypothalamus axis can function poorly when it is irrigated insufficiently. Cranial Osteopaths have long established that children born with forceps, or Ventouse delivery and those with head and neck injuries at birth, or later, develop eczema, asthma and are generally very 'chesty', with frequent colds and coughs. Their immune system is poor. Gentle Cranio-Sacral work establishes good flow of the CSF and the Pituitary-Hypothalamus also gets additional nutrition. This cures such problems.

A clinical trial carried out in a leading London Hospital showed that Cranial Osteopathy helped to change immunological markers in blood for the better.

> My techniques, which are more to do with blood than CSF circulation in that area, showed remarkable results. In 1994, I gathered case histories of some twenty-five children and went to meet Dr Andrew Bush at the Royal Brompton Hospital. He was a consultant in Respiratory Disease. I explained my technique of diet, neck massage and yogic breathing exercise for the treatment of Asthma. He was very impressed, but the research committee found the approach too anecdotal and opted to fund a different trial using complimentary medicine. Medical science apparently cannot accept that such a safe and effective treatment can help a serious condition like asthma. 'Where is the catch?' they ask.

Later in this book I will discuss another case where, years later, Professor Andrew Bush was completely taken aback by a beautiful 3 year old Russian girl having her life saved by these techniques only to lose it later during a complicated surgery.

2. Adaptation

This is a unique phenomenon in all living beings. The Hypothalamus assesses the changes in the environment and brings about physiological and emotional adjustments so that the body and the mind can cope with the situation.

If you go to a hot and sunny place, fair skin acquires a tan within hours. The bright sun can damage the skin and the pigment melanin helps to block it.

If you go to an altitude, the lack of oxygen makes you breathe differently until such time when the bone marrow produces more haemoglobin and Red Blood Cells. If you are at 2,000 metres, a healthy body may take two days to adjust. If you go above 3,000 metres, you may need five days to adapt.

I have led treks in the higher Himalayas over the past twenty years. In the beginning, we experienced a lot of complications, such as pounding headaches, altered breathing – faster and faster at first and then at the peak breathing stops for a few seconds and then start all over again. This is called Cheyne-Stokes breathing. In sleep Apnoea, a condition that sounds very scary to a companion, a similar breathing pattern is noticed. Those who go into a coma have similar breathing, but nowadays ventilators change the breathing artificially.

One year, I took to the trek my therapists, who gave us all an hour's massage. It took much less time to adapt as my technique was applied to improve the blood flow to the brain. Now we have made it a standard feature for each group, so nausea, panic attacks and fainting are a thing of the past.

On winding mountain roads, those with neck problems also get motion sickness and they are asked to fix their eyes on one spot at a time. It is a pity because the scenery is so magnificent.

3. Homeostasis (homeo – unchanging; statis – standing)

This is a phenomenon in the body that maintains harmony. The pH of the blood is a constant 7.4. You may drink a litre of lemon juice, but the blood will be automatically alkalised so that the pH value remains the same. The cells function optimally at that pH level (7 is normal and 7.4 is slightly alkaline).

The level of blood cells, sugar, protein, salts, cholesterol, uric acid, body temperature, heart rate, breathing rate, day-night cycle etc are all kept in harmony within certain ranges. Nature knows that cells function optimally in a certain environment, so it works around the clock to maintain that balance or harmony through the Hypothalamus-Pituitary system. Normal blood tests are results of our Homeostosis functioning well.

If, for example, some bacteria or viruses enter the body, in a defensive tactic the thermostat in the hypothalamus is adjusted to raise the body temperature so that the invading organisms cannot thrive. They too like a cosy environment. The use of Paracetamol, however, instructs the sweat glands to open and secrete. The sweat evaporates on the skin and the body temperature, or fever, falls to its near-normal level. This is an example of sacrificing the natural cure for the sake of comfort.

Homeostasis is absolutely essential for our survival. This is the pillar that supports the Innate Healing Power. The disease process, or pathogenic force, overcomes the health process, or sanogenic forces, to cause an illness. Homeostasis, an arm of the Innate Healing Power, re-harmonises the body's chemistry and immune system, to bring them back to the optimum level in order to create health.

The Pituitary Gland secretes hormones that control the functions of vital organs and systems; the thyroid gland, the adrenal glands, the reproductive system, blood sugar regulation, growth, etc.

1. The Thyroid Gland

This is the body's main regulator of metabolism (total chemical processes). Its hormone, Thyroxine, production is stimulated by the Pituitary, via the hormone, appropriately called the Thyroid Stimulating Hormone (TSH). Lack of Thyroxine production is commonly called 'low thyroid', which is known as Hypothyroidism (Hypo- low). When that happens the metabolic rate (the 'burning' of fuel in the cells to produce energy) slows down. There is cellulite, or white fat accumulation on the body, swelling of the body, intolerance to heat, slow motivation, which makes you lazy, with dry skin, low body temperature, hair loss, menstrual problems, chronic fatigue, depression, body aches etc. It is as if there is a 'power failure' in the body and nothing works.

As iodine is an essential element in the production of Thyroxine, any such deficiency in the diet often leads to Hypothyroidism. Those who believe in Natural Medicine, therefore, take Sea Kelp, which is rich in Iodine to help Hypothyroidism.

Sometimes the opposite happens and the thyroid gland produces excess

Thyroxine. That causes an increase in the metabolic rate. The skin is flushed, it is moist with sweat, the heart rate increases often causing irregular beats, the blood pressure increases as a result, there is anxiety, tremor in the hands' many suffer diarrhoea, weight loss, insomnia etc. In spite of high excitation in the body, the person feels shattered and cannot function. This condition is called 'overactive thyroid' or Hyperthyroidism. In this case the Pituitary is not the main cause. There is often a tumour in the thyroid gland called'goitre' with hyperactive cells producing excess Thyroxine.

Hypothyroidism is generally caused by lack of stimulation from the Pituitary gland through Thyroid Stimulating Hormone (TSH). This malfunction is triggered by reduced blood supply to that area.

There is another type of hormone called Calcitonin which is secreted by the deeper tissues of the thyroid. The cells that produce this are called' C' Cells ('C' is for clear). Calcitonin reduces the calcium level in the blood by stimulating its excretion by the kidneys and suppressing the bone cells so that they don't release calcium into the blood.

Behind the thyroid gland is a pair of glands called the Parathyroid Glands. These glands, which are very small in size, secrete parathyroid hormones which increase the level of calcium in the blood. This effect is the opposite of that of Calcitonin. An overactive parathyroid gland can stimulate the release of calcium from the bones and cause osteoporosis. The bone supply calcium to the blood in this case.

It is interesting how the complex of the different glands in the thyroid region aid muscular activity, to either increase or decrease energy production. Calcium stimulates muscle contraction and so energy is lost, whilst its inhibition will increase energy production.

We still do not know how the thyroid's 'C' cells and Parathyroid glands are regulated, but we can positively guess that such a delicate job like balancing calcium in the blood can only be carried out by the Hypothalamus-Pituitary axis.

2. The Adrenal Glands

These are a yellow pyramid-shaped pair of gland that sits on the kidneys. They are only 7.5 grammes in weight, but their action on the body is powerful. The yellow colour is due to the presence of stored lipids, or fat molecules, like cholesterol and fatty acids, the raw material for production of the adrenal hormones in the cortex, or outer layer of the adrenal gland. These hormones are collectively known as corticosteroids (these are 'steroids' found naturally in the body). So vital are these corticosteroids for the body that if the glands are removed, the body will die unless they are replaced by artificial steroids (the very hormones we are all conscious of).

The outer layer of the adrenal gland produces aldosterone, a hormone that controls minerals in the body – the two most important of these minerals are sodium and potassium. The functions of nerves, muscles, kidneys, sweat gland, salivary glands, digestive enzyme secretion in the intestines etc, are controlled by the balance of sodium and potassium levels in both tissue fluid and blood. Thus, if blood pressure drops or there is loss of blood, the sodium level drops. This releases the mineral regulator Aldosterone and the loss of fluid through the kidneys, sweat, saliva etc are immediately controlled in order to maintain optimum levels in the blood. This is one example of how homeostasis works.

The middle thicker layer of the adrenal cortex synthesises and secretes Glucocorticoids like Hydrocortisone and cortisone. These are popularly known as 'corticoids. The Pituitary secretes ACTH, a hormone that stimulates the Adrenal Cortex (middle layer) to secrete Cortisone and Hydrocortisone. These cortisols are also the day hormones that keep us functioning during the day.

These hormones synthesise glucose (glycogen) in the liver. The hydrocortisone in the blood helps control inflammation of joints and tissues etc. That is why artificial steroid creams are used for eczema or skin rashes. It suppresses the activity of the immune cells. Artificial steroids are used for suppressing asthma, hives, rheumatoid arthritis, psoriasis etc.

Use of artificial steroids confuses the Hypothalamus and it begins to think that the adrenal cortex is functioning well, so it stops further stimulation. The cells of the adrenal cortex become lazy and can atrophy from lack of stimulation. This amounts to the total loss of functions of the adrenal cortex and one needs to be artificially stimulated. Steroids are 'emergency' hormones and should not be circulating in the blood all the time. Artificial steroids have many side-effects like osteoporosis, weakening of the defences of the immune system, damage to the liver and kidneys, swellings on the body (especially the face) etc. Thus, steroids should be administered with extreme caution.

The innermost layer of the adrenal gland secretes androgens, or male hormones, similar to testosterone. If it is overactive in women they may develop muscles, grow a beard, lose hair on the scalp, deposit cellulite on the arms and thighs, have large breasts etc especially if the ovaries have cysts and fail to convert testosterone into oestrogen.

Excess androgen (DHEA, male hormones) is unwanted in a female body. It is converted or aromatized by fat cells into a female hormone ESTERONE, which is deposited as cellulite (white non-dietary, soft, with a cottage-cheese texture) in specific areas. These areas lie below the belly-button to resemble early pregnancy; something most women hate, around the waist, from the hip down to the knee on the thighs, from the shoulder to the elbow and in the breast. The cellulite spares the face and other parts of the body.

This esterone can also be produced in men due to a crisis of mistaken identity; In this case men develop breasts and have the body shape of a woman with cellulite (fat thighs, lower belly, fat arms etc). Many teenagers suffer from this condition in puberty. These boys get such a complex as peers tease them about their breasts. They stop swimming, lock doors when changing clothes, shun T-shirts that may divulge their breasts etc.

Prolonged stress in women leads to hyperstimulation of the adrenal cortex by the hypothalamus-pituitary, leading to the cellulite deposits. These women control their diet, eat sparingly and try their best to avoid fats and sugar, but the weight just keeps increasing. I have written about this type of weight gain (Hormonal Weight Gain) in my book 'Dr Ali's Weight loss Plan' and 'Dr Ali's Woman's Health Bible'.

The innermost part of the adrenal gland secretes adrenaline (epinephrine) and nor adrenaline (norepinephrine). There is always some amount of these hormones secreted in the blood to keep us going, if there is an emergency or stressful situation and the body needs a heightened response, the hypothalamus stimulates this part, via the sympathetic nervous system. Large amounts of adrenaline are secreted in the blood. Stored glucose in the liver and muscles is released to produce extra energy. The heart rate, breathing rate, tension in the muscles and the metabolic rate increase to create the classic 'fight' or flight' reaction.

When a fox sees a rabbit, its adrenaline prepares it for a fight, or chase, whilst the rabbit in fear also under the influence of the same hormone, is ready for flight. The emotions are different, but the body's reaction is the same.

If a stressful situation continues for days or months, the adrenaline secretion is constant. The body is in a permanent state of alertness and anxiety, as if it is fighting a running battle. This exhausts the body and there is an ultimate breakdown of the hypothalamic control system. This manifests into short or long-term illness like high blood pressure, auto-immune disease, psychological conditions, IBS, cancer etc.

3. The Reproductive system

The main Pituitary hormones, that stimulate testicular tissue in males and ovarian tissue in females, are FSH (Follicle Stimulating Hormone) and LH (Luteinising Hormone). These increase the production of Testosterone in males.

In females, these hormones first mature the 'follicles' or cells that contain egg cells. The most matured follicle releases a single egg and 'ovulation' takes place. The empty follicle then begins to secrete progesterone, which prepares the uterine lining to receive a potentially fertilized egg. The lining of the uterus thickens and if the egg is not fertilised within their 4-5 day lifespan, then the progesterone prepares to break up the uterine lining and the period starts. Thus, the menstrual cycle and fertility of women are controlled by the Hypothalamus-Pituitary axis.

4. Blood Sugar Regulation

The Pancreas has a dual function. It secretes pancreatic juice that digests protein, fats and carbohydrates in the intestines. The other function is that it regulates blood sugar, by means of insulin and glucagon secretion in the blood. While insulin uses-up excess glucose by sweeping it off into the cells, glucagon releases more glucose by breaking-down stored chemicals in the liver and muscles. These two hormones have contradicting functions and yet the cells that produce them are neighbours.

Again, this is a perfect example of homeostatis or the self-regulatory phenomenon that maintains harmony and equilibrium in the body. The Hypothalamus has an indirect, or direct, role in maintaining the balance. When the system breaks-up, as in Diabetes, the insulin production is either inadequate, or the cells of the body are too damaged to allow insulin to prepare them to accept glucose. When insulin is insufficient, because the pancreatic cells don't produce it, Type I, or Insulin Dependent Diabetes sets in. If the glucose utilization by cells is poor, even though enough insulin is produced, then the result is excess blood sugar and this is called Type II Diabetes.

In this case the cell-walls are either damaged by free-radicals or overworked due to excessive consumption of sugar and alcohol.

5. Growth

Although the Pituitary secretes the Growth Hormone until around twenty-one years of age, other hormones such as Insulin, Thyroxin, Cortisol from the adrenals, reproductive hormones like Testosterone and Oestrogen, especially during puberty, also help growth and repair of cells. Pituitary Growth Hormone helps the skeletal system to grow. Many adults who are short in height have a history of birth or other head and neck injury before puberty.

Excess Growth Hormone can boost height at puberty. Many teenagers suffer from growing pains. The bone shafts and spine grow rapidly and the attached muscles cannot cope. This results in, often, excruciating pain in muscle tendons in the groin, knees, Achilles tendon etc.

Hormones can affect moods. Those who take steroids know how agitated they feel. They cannot relax or sleep very well. At puberty, the surge of reproductive hormones makes teenagers very hyperactive, aggressive, unreasonable, hyper energetic etc.

Hormones can contribute to premature ageing. The levels of Thyroid, water regulatory hormones, cortisol, adrenaline etc. remain unchanged with age. The insulin production may decrease, however, and this results in the elderly getting late-onset Diabetes. The Growth Hormone levels decrease and so repair work, muscle and bone building capacity drop. Thus, the elderly are more likely to develop muscle atrophy and osteoporosis.

Finally, the importance of the Hypothalamus- Pituitary- axis is demonstrated by the anatomy of the blood vessels (See Fig. 3). The two vertebral arteries join at the base of the Pons (Top of the brain stem) to form a single Basilar Artery (Base artery). This artery bifurcates above the Pons and circles around the Pituitary. This ring of blood vessels, called the Circle of Willis, gets some additional blood from the Internal Carotid which is another artery that mostly feeds the conscious brain. Having lost blood to its various branches in the subconscious brain, its level drops and it gets some fresh supply from a neighbour, so that the Hypothalamus-Pituitary gets ample blood. This boost in blood supply indicates that this area of the brain needs maximum and constant supply. The manufacture of hormones and coordinating functions of the body require extra energy. This is, after all, the Headquarters of the body's autonomous nervous system.

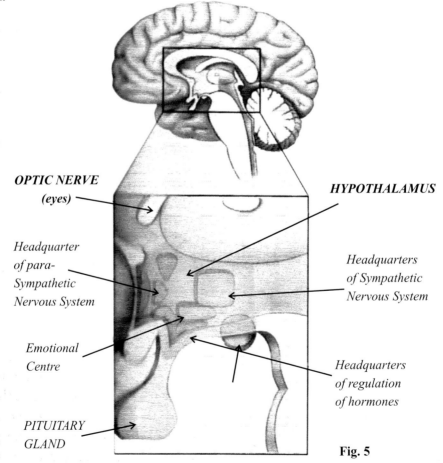

OPTIC NERVE
(eyes)

HYPOTHALAMUS

Headquarter of para-Sympathetic Nervous System

Headquarters of Sympathetic Nervous System

Emotional Centre

Headquarters of regulation of hormones

PITUITARY GLAND

Fig. 5

Section of the Brain showing location of Pituitary Gland, Hypothalamus, Emotional

Another clever invention of Nature is that the Pituitary and other glands secrete their hormones into the venous system. This way they bypass the minute capillaries which lie at the end of the arteries. The veins carry the hormones quickly to the heart and then to the rest of the body. Thus the Vertebral Veins, located in the vertebral canals, are just as important as their accompanying arteries. They carry important hormones to the heart. Thus, obstruction to the blood-flow through these veins in the vertebral canal, or the neck area, has a serious effect on our health. These hormones of the brain (melatonin, ACTH, TSH, FSH, ADH) are vital messengers.

The Pons

This part of the brain houses the nuclei, or nerve centres, of several important cranial nerves. Lack of blood supply to the roots of these nerves, through tiny blood vessels called vasa nervorum (vas – vessels) or to the Pons directly, can cause:

- Bells' Palsy when one side of the face is paralysed, the eyes are wide open, the angle of the mouth drops

- Lack of coordination of the eye muscles and sometimes double-vision.

- Tinnitus when the auditory nerve or its centre in the Pons does not get enough blood.

- Irregular breathing as in high altitude, panic attacks, coma etc.

- Trigeminal neuralgia which is a serious painful disease affecting one half of the face or jaw or forehead. The Trigeminal Nerve has 3 branches (tri-three)

The Cerebellum

There is a pair of arteries on each side of the Cerebellum that branch off the vertebral-basilar arteries. It is therefore well nourished. Although the function of the Cerebellum is not wholly understood, there is evidence that it is the main centre of coordination. We know that gait, posture, and balance are controlled from here. Besides these, perhaps other forms of coordination like playing music, singing, speaking, writing, driving, riding a bicycle etc must also be coordinated from here.

I have seen several patients who have had a stroke of the cerebellum. Their balance was severely affected and they suffered dizziness.

Increasingly excessive stress, computer use, trauma etc, neck injury or the tightness of muscles, impair blood flow to the cerebellum. Dizziness and nausea are therefore becoming more common. Even vertigo is becoming a recognisable medical condition. Most doctors blame the inner ear for it and often call it 'Meniere's Disease'. I have, however, successfully treated it with my technique, which should prove the cerebellum's blood supply was the culprit. A classic Meniere's disease is dizziness accompanied by tinnitus. I hope some doctors will read this and revise their opinion. I would, of course, understand the diagnosis if there were a problem with a tumour in the inner ear, or some structural fault after injury. Sometimes, 'crystals' in the inner ear may cause vertigo or dizziness.

The Medulla Oblongata

This part of the brain connects the brain with the spinal cord. It has numerous nerve fibres connecting the brain with the rest of the body below.

This part controls the heart rate, strength of its contraction, and the circulation in smaller blood vessels. The rhythm and depth of respiration is controlled from here in conjunction with corresponding centres in the Pons.

It also has centres that control digestive juice secretion, the movement of food through the gut, swallowing, movement of vocal cords etc.

It is nourished by vertebral arteries and receives the blood it requires, unless there is a major obstruction. As the arteries progress up to the higher parts of the brain, they distribute blood all along, loosing volume gradually. Thus, the higher vital centres can be more affected because of neck problems.

Difficulties in swallowing and severe digestive problems are extreme complications of reduced blood flow through vertebral arteries.

To sum up, The Ali Syndrome is a complex concept which involves understanding the inner sanctums of the brain, so it is not surprising it has evaded scientific explanation so far and is only now becoming clear as brain research advances. Its diagnosis is equally hard to comprehend and is therefore the subject of the next chapter.

Diagnosing the Ali Syndrome

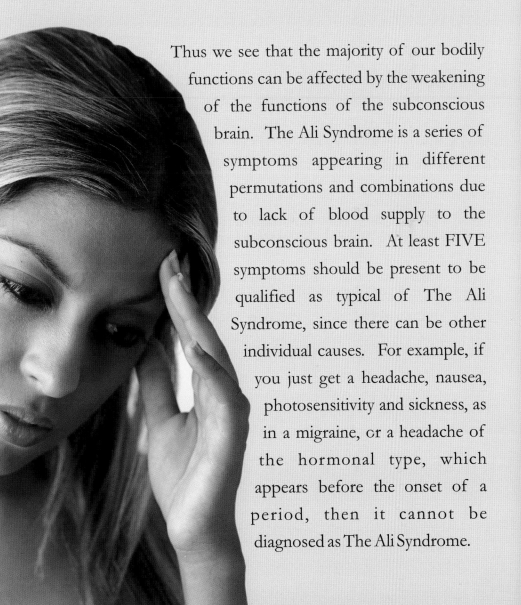

Thus we see that the majority of our bodily functions can be affected by the weakening of the functions of the subconscious brain. The Ali Syndrome is a series of symptoms appearing in different permutations and combinations due to lack of blood supply to the subconscious brain. At least FIVE symptoms should be present to be qualified as typical of The Ali Syndrome, since there can be other individual causes. For example, if you just get a headache, nausea, photosensitivity and sickness, as in a migraine, or a headache of the hormonal type, which appears before the onset of a period, then it cannot be diagnosed as The Ali Syndrome.

In a case of Chronic Fatigue Syndrome, however, with symptoms like fatigue, muzzy head, headaches, sleep disturbances (jet-lag type sleep), dizziness, short-term memory loss, lack of concentration, depression, lack of motivation, craving for sugar, palpitation, panic attacks, a poor immune system, cold hands and feet etc, then The Ali Syndrome can be diagnosed. In fact, a typical CFS is almost certainly The Ali Syndrome if trauma to the head and neck precede the onset of these symptoms. It is essential to establish that the lack of blood flow to the subconscious brain, due to the conditions of the neck mentioned earlier, has been the primary cause. For example, if you get viral infections, such as Epstein Barr or other viruses, then the same symptoms may also prevail (as in ME) when it is not The Ali Syndrome: The neck has to be involved in the case.

The most common symptoms of the Ali Syndrome are chronic fatigue, headaches, a jet-lag type sleep pattern, and short- term memory loss, craving for sugar, lack of concentration, tinnitus and neck tension. On physical examination of the neck, one should find tender points on one or the other side of the neck. If probed carefully, some protrusions can be found along the side of the vertebrae. These hard 'lumps' are sore to touch. The protrusions are due to misaligned cervical vertebrae and are in actual fact displaced wings (transverse process). Such displacement is more common at the level of the 3rd or 4th vertebra. Sometimes pressing on these protrusions can cause a headache on the corresponding side. This may sometimes cause tinnitus (a loud noise in the ear).

If the person is asked to move the head sideways towards the left and right shoulder for 5-10 times, he, or she, will experience dizziness to some degree. In severe displacement of the vertebrae, the dizziness will be more pronounced. Sometimes, this causes some degree of nausea, blurred vision and imbalance. This is a universal test for The Ali Syndrome. The dizziness caused by movement of the neck is an indication that there is an obstruction of the blood flow to the Cerebellum, caused by misalignment in the neck. One may argue that this could be an inner ear problem. In order to exclude that, I ask the person to bend the head forward and backward for 5-10 times to its maximum point. If there is dizziness, then the inner ear is the cause. Lateral movement puts maximum pressure on the arteries and this reduces the blood flow even further.

It is best to go through the checklist for a range of symptoms that constitute The Ali Syndrome. The more positive symptoms there are, the more sure you can be that you have the syndrome.

Some other, less convincing, tests are soreness in the area of the occiput, in the back of the skull, where the tendons of the neck muscles are attached. Further questioning may be necessary: Do you feel fatigue or dizziness in a crowded place, like the metro or a crowded bar, in a smoky environment, when you are in steam room, or when you inhale petrol fumes or wet paint? Do you feel sick when driving on winding country roads? Do you sleep with the windows open and keep your face out of the duvet or blanket?

Do you feel clear-headed when you are in fresh air? Does mountain air make you less tired or dizzy or sick? Have you had an accident, birth injury or whiplash?

All the above questions can confirm that reduced oxygen supply to the brain makes the symptoms more intense. Stagnant air makes you worse, whilst fresh air makes you feel better.

Another relevant question is 'Do you feel tired and sleepy immediately after a meal?' If blood flow to the brain is already restricted, the formation of a blood depot around the stomach and intestines after meals deprives the subconscious brain of more blood/oxygen. This causes extreme fatigue and dizziness.

A similar situation occurs just before a period when there is pelvic congestion. Women have worse PMS (Premenstrual Syndrome) when they have neck problems and when they suffer from The Ali Syndrome.

The following conditions make the symptoms of the Ali Syndrome more pronounced:

- Dehydration (reduces blood volume)
- Anaemia (reduces Haemoglobin or iron)
- Low blood pressure
- Excessive sweating (causes loss of salt)
- Candida infection in the gut, which produces toxic alcohol in the gut and so there is already an underlying fatigue
- The use of recreational drugs or excessive alcohol consumption
- Altitude
- Chronic diarrhoea
- Osteoporosis
- Deficiency of hormones, including thyroxine, testosterone, oestrogen (as in menopause)
- Diabetes
- Chronic underlying illnesses such as cancer

Self Diagnosis

One can self-diagnose The Ali Syndrome. When I used to write a weekly column in the YOU magazine with the Mail on Sunday, I used to mention The Ali Syndrome. Some doctors criticised me by email but those patients who suffered from it could easily identify the cluster of core symptoms that go together as a complex. I often had patients who would come to me and say 'I think I have got the Ali Syndrome.'

In 'Dr Ali's Ultimate Back Book', published in 2002, I wrote a chapter called 'The Neck Connection', referring to my discovery. This book sold many copies and I had patients with The Ali Syndrome saying 'it seems you have described my illness.' It is an accurate assessment of this condition.

To summarize, here is a comprehensive list of the symptoms which constitute The Ali Syndrome:

- Chronic fatigue
- Breathlessness
- Headaches, both general or one-sided
- Dizziness or vertigo
- Nausea
- Sickness with vomiting
- Palpitation (an increased heart rate)
- Hyperventilation (breathlessness)
- Panic attacks, which are a combination of the two previous symptoms
- Cravings for carbohydrates - sugar in particular
- Short-term memory loss
- Jet-lag type sleep patterns (awake at night and tired during the day)
- Lack of concentration and often absent-mindedness
- Lack of comprehension (feeling 'blank')
- Tinnitus (ringing in the ears)
- Weak immune system with frequent coughs and colds
- Allergic reactions (Eczema, asthma)
- Asymmetry of the face
- Autoimmune Disease, including Rheumatoid Arthritis, Psoriasis, Lupus
- Extreme intolerance to white wine and Champagne
- Rosacea (redness in the cheeks)
- Mellasma (dark pigmentation on the face or skin)

- Bells Palsy
- Trigeminal Neuralgia
- Blurred vision or loss of field vision (some)
- Polymyalgia Rheumatica(auto-immune disease)
- Food intolerances
- Retarded growth in teenagers
- Amenorrhoea (lack of periods)
- Aggravated menopausal symptoms (hot flushes, anxiety)
- Unexplained infertility
- Nervous tic on the face
- Post-herpetic burning in the face, neck, torso
- Burning sensation in the arms , thighs, feet (sympathetic nervous Dystopia)
- Burning mouth syndrome
- Accentuated smell (strong smell)
- Depression (not clinical depression ,which is a Disease)
- Double vision
- Loss of the sense of smell or taste after an accident or trauma
- Burning mouth syndrome (on the tongue and palate)
- Loss of libido and Impotence
- Irregular periods
- Loss of periods after stress, trauma or a whiplash injury
- Polycystic Ovarian Syndrome
- Premature Puberty (before 10 years of age)
- Cold hands and feet and also chilblains
- Blotchy skin
- Globus Hystericus ('lump' in the throat due to anxiety)
- Fainting - in extreme cases (syncope)
- Bruxism (grinding teeth whilst asleep)
- Sleep Apnoea (intermittent breathing)
- Restless legs at night
- Narcolepsy (abnormally long sleep)
- Reynaud's Syndrome (white glove-like hands which are freezing cold)
- Hypersensitive skin on one side of the face or arms
- Water Retention
- Fatigue after meals and PMS or PMT
- Imbalance
- Car or motion sickness
- Mild Hypertension (Blood Pressure)
- Weight gain
- Macular degeneration (loss of vision due to age or after accidents)
- Cerebral palsy
- Epileptic fits after head and neck injury
- Possibly Autism, Dyslexia if related to birth injuries

If there is a Hypothalamic malfunction, there is a test that can be used to prove it. Take a blunt tipped object, such as a used biro, paper cutter, the blunt end of a thick needle sterilize with spirit if you have at home and scratch two parallel lines on the inner surface of the forearm. Wait for a few seconds. If the scratch lines turn red, then everything is fine. However, if it is pale and does not turn red in a minute, then the Hypothalamus, which is the controller of the tone of smaller blood vessels, is malfunctioning. The pressure on the blood vessels under the skin flattens them, hence the pale colour. Normally, the vessels will spring back and dilate to allow more blood through a natural reflex action. The lines turn red. If the capillaries fail to respond and go into spasm, then they turn pale and this is indicative of a lack of a message from the Hypothalamus.

Sometimes, there is an abnormal response after a couple of minutes. The two scratch lines remain very pale but on either side the blood vessels dilate. Thus you see four red lines and two pale lines. This is also due to an abnormal response from the circulatory control system of the Hypothalamus.

This test is termed 'positive' when the scratch lines remain pale. It means that parts of the Hypothalamus and indeed the Sympathetic Nervous System, (the Autonomous or involuntary nervous system) are not functioning very well.

This is an indirect way of proving the malfunction of the subconscious brain, which causes The Ali Syndrome. Visual proof with blotchy pink 'marble' like skin on the arms is another telltale sign. The blood vessels constrict or dilate under the skin to create this 'blotchy' look. Then you can touch the left and right half of the skull or face. If one side feels more sensitive than the other, then the presence of the symptoms of The Ali Syndrome is very likely. This difference in sensation is probably due to the lack of blood flow to the root of the 5th cranial (Trigeminal) Nerve. The roots are thick and are fed by tiny blood vessels of the Basilar-Vertebral arteries. This is the sensory nerve for the face and part of the scalp.

If the person with the Ali Syndrome is emotional, or enters a warm stuffy room, the cheeks turn pink. The Hypothalamus mistakenly 'thinks 'that the body is over-heated and so sends instructions to dilate blood vessels, which are plenty in the cheek area, to radiate heat.

Variations in symptoms

The million-dollar question is why some symptoms of The Ali Syndrome are more prominent or noticeable than others? As I mentioned before, reduced blood volume decreases its pressure and depending on the genetically controlled anatomy of the various blood vessels, some areas are more starved than others. Then there is this phenomenon of the 'Law of Dominance', as I call it. If you have several damaged root canals in the teeth, the worst of them will hurt first. One strong symptom will dominate the others. If you have vertigo, the chances are you will feel nauseous, anxious and panicky but your pain will be suppressed. The body likes to deal with a few symptoms at a time. Some symptoms such as low thyroid, poor immunity, rheumatoid arthritis, etc may gradually manifest themselves over a period of time.

People have varying threshold levels for pain, discomfort, dizziness, depression etc. Strong-minded people, or those who have very demanding or responsible jobs, tend to override their symptoms more easily. Some have a 'Get on with it' attitude to life. It's when a headache is noticeable and vertigo, or imbalance, which makes them lose confidence that they take notice and seek a doctor's help. If one gets Bell's Palsy (paralysis of one half of the face), then one is very alarmed.

Acute or Chronic?

Although most symptoms of the Ali Syndrome are chronic, or manifest themselves over a period of time, an acute attack can also happen. Vaso-vagal Reaction is one of them. An acute or sudden loss of blood supply to the subconscious brain can cause a person to have a black-out and faint. Such patients even see the 'shrouding darkness' coming just before fainting, though they often don't remember this. Acute dehydration, a crowded place, hot sun, sudden stress from the delivery of bad news, etc can trigger this reaction. You just have to lay the sufferer flat on their back, massage the neck gently and stretch it and they will revive. A drink of water or sweetened juice will replenish the energy supply to the brain.

The most intolerable symptoms of The Ali Syndrome are Cluster Headaches, (very painful headaches that recur frequently) especially when you get them every day, all of the time for three months or so and vertigo, when you sway to one side and collapse as the world around you spins in one or the other direction. You have total loss of control. My technique has come to the rescue of many such patients.

Exclusions

The symptoms I have mentioned are the most common ones associated with The Ali Syndrome. There are many symptoms which have been excluded in the above list. The subconscious brain regulates everything in the body and so many more symptoms are found. Hypoglycaemia (drop in blood sugar), autoimmune diseases such as Vitiligo, alopecia, Schogren's (with dry saliva and eyes etc), Parkinsonism, essential tremors (in the hands and head) etc have been deliberately excluded because I have not been successful in curing them using my techniques which, amongst other things, improve blood and CSF flow to the Subconscious Brain.

Often, damage occurs in Parkinson's syndrome where brain cells die in the *substantia nigra* part of the brain that produces dopamine (a nerve stimulator) and the body's coordination system fails. This causes tremors in the lips, head, hands and arms, loss of facial expression and difficulty in starting an activity. Once started, walking or getting up, the person can go on doing it. These specialized *substantia nigra* (black substance) fail and probably change irreversibly, so irrigating that area with blood does not revive them.

So far I have presented the Ali Syndrome in a manner similar to the general approach to any medical condition. This one, however, tends to be so much more diverse that I feel that my experience in mastering it may give a better idea of the extent to which it needs to be explored to gain a full understanding of its scope. In the next chapter I will approach it more from my own experience rather than follow a strict analysis of its appearance, cause, diagnosis and treatment.

Exploring the Ali Syndrome

The Ali Syndrome is best understood by examining its major symptoms and parallel influences on the body, particularly in cases which I have treated, in one case myself.

6.1 Chronic Fatigue Syndrome (CFS)

CFS is probably the most classic example of The Ali Syndrome. It can display many of the symptoms mentioned earlier. I call this 'the Power Failure of the body'. It's as if someone has turned down the life force. Besides fatigue, the main symptom, there is an entire range of symptoms such as headaches, dizziness, nausea, lack of motivation, short-term memory loss, jet-lag sleep, lack of concentration, a 'muzzy' or 'foggy' head, as if you are absorbed in a TV programme and you are not in the world around you, loss of libido, dysfunctional periods in women, body-ache from loss of muscle tone, palpitation, a poor immune system. One has to have 80% of the above symptoms to be classified as a sufferer of CFS>

When one is run down and the immune system weakens, one is likely to contract a virus called Epstein Barr (the Glandular Fever virus). The virus attacks lymph nodes and power cells (called mitochondria) in muscle tissues. This condition is called ME (Myalgic Encephalomyelitis), otherwise known as Post-viral Fatigue. In this case, extreme muscle ache and intense fatigue are the main symptoms. Other symptoms of CFS mentioned above may also be present as the viral infection also affects the brain tissue, including that of the subconscious brain. Neck tension is also an absolute symptom of ME.

Since a poor immune system, caused by neck tension and exhaustion, precedes the viral infection, ME is also regarded as a complication of the Ali Syndrome. It is an extension of CFS. Therefore, CFS and ME are treated with similar therapies.   Since ME is a post-viral fatigue, the antiviral treatment is not recommended. The infection has gone but has left behind a total mess. When the storm passes the devastation remains.

6.2 Effects of Altitude

I have been using my techniques at an altitude of up to 2000metres to treat CFS and other conditions for the past 22 years or so. Sportsmen and army personnel often train at altitude to improve their stamina.   The results obtained after the treatment of CFS patients at altitude is even more convincing. Firstly, patients adapt to a different environment, culture, food, sounds, colours, and the people of the Himalayan region.   Then the body has to adapt to the altitude.   Although up to 2000 metres, one doesn't have the usual side-effects of altitude of over 2500metres, when one gets tired, dizzy, insomnia, palpitation, imbalance, headaches etc.   At this intermediate altitude, the body is put through some stress but there are no uncomfortable symptoms.

Patients with CFS go through a programme of yoga, walking for 2-4 hours in the valley or mountains, diet and most importantly, my massage technique.   The walks are graded so that one walks on different gradients, or for longer, each day. The fatigue from walking and aches caused by the strain on the joints and lactic acid in the muscles is eliminated through massage.   One therefore feels fresh each morning.   In the morning the yoga asanas refresh the mind and invigorate the body.   This programme is done over a period of ten days or so.   The patients notice the change in their condition and become more confident.   Some walk additionally in the evening and continue to feel very energetic.   This helps to remove the burden of being tired all the time.   This new found energy creates a very positive 'feel-good' factor.

In the late '80's when I started this altitude therapy, I carried out blood tests before and after treatment. The average increase in Haemoglobin levels was 0.5gms and there was an increase in Red Blood Cells. At high altitude, the body needs more oxygen as its supply in the air is reduced. The yoga and walking forces the body to produce more haemoglobin in the blood, so more oxygen can be supplied to the tissues. The neck treatment improves the blood supply to the subconscious brain. This creates the 'feel-good' factor, which improves energy levels and the immune system.

Pollution in cities and urban areas lengthens the treatment of CFS. In fact, patients treated at altitude feel very tired for a few days after returning to polluted places. Then, after adaptation, the energy comes back. This is when they are encouraged to go to the gym, walk in fresh air or to spend weekends in hilly places. The benefits achieved at altitude stabilize and the body heals itself in a few weeks. This is how CFS sufferers are rehabilitated in their mind and body.

This is a clear-cut proof that improving blood flow, which increases oxygen and glucose supply to the brain, re-energises the body and mind. This helps the subconscious brain function better and stimulates the Innate Healing Power, the precursor to elimination of symptoms of illness and the creation of wellbeing.

6.3 PET Scans

There is a special type of investigation called a PET (Positron Emission Tomography) scan, where radioactive glucose is injected in the blood and then a series of photos are taken to see how they are distributed. If a part of the brain, or body, doesn't receive enough blood, the concentration of this glucose, in those particular tissues, will be reduced.

In California, PET scans of the brain were done in patients with CFS. It showed hypo-perfusion (reduced supply) of blood in the brain tissue in over 65% of cases. The results published did not specify whether the subconscious part of the brain was more affected in patients who showed these positive findings. I am confident that if such a study were repeated, my hypothesis could be proved.

PET scans are expensive and uncomfortable, as the head needs to be fixed for imaging. Sometimes the scans may take a long time to do and that is disturbing for those who are claustrophobic and have to go into a machine. Never-the-less, it remains a concrete method of proving that lack of blood supply to the brain is one of the contributing factors of CFS.

6.4 Headaches

I will have to specify that under this heading all headaches, except for migraine, will be covered. All migraines are headaches but not all headaches are migraines. This type of headache is an illness which involves vomiting, sensitivity to light or sound, intense half-sided headaches which last for 2-3days before settling down on their own and is periodic in nature, occurring in women just before menstruation begins.

Headache is a symptom which can be caused by various factors. The most common cause is the impaired blood flow to the brain due to neck problems. All osteopaths and chiropractors will also confirm this because, within seconds of neck manipulation, the patient will be relieved of a headache. This happens in the vast majority of cases.

6.5 Non-Ali Syndrome Headaches

There are categories of headaches which do not respond to the therapy that improves blood flow to the brain. These causes of headaches are not related to the neck. If one has a frontal, or forehead, headache, it is most likely to be due to sinus congestion. You may have a clear nose, but the sinuses are packed with thick mucus which may occasionally drip down the throat. This is termed 'Post Nasal Drip'. To treat it you have to avoid mucus producing foods, such as dairy, ice creams, sorbets etc. My sinus oil, containing sesame, mustard and eucalyptus oils, dropped into the nostrils and sniffed, helps to de-congest 'blocked' sinuses. The headache then disappears.

If one clenches the jaw, grinds one teeth at night, eats a lot of nuts or hard meat, one is likely to get arthritis, or inflammation, of the jaw joint (TMJ – temporomandibular joint)) located in front of the ear. This joint becomes very sore to touch. The pain from this joint can irradiate to the temples and mimic a one-sided headache. It is often confused with the half-sided neck type of headaches experienced by the majority of sufferers. Massage the affected joint, with some balm or oil, for a few minutes a day and the headaches will disappear almost instantly after the massage.

Headaches due to High Blood Pressure are usually felt in the back of the head in the occiput area. Treat the BP problem and the headache disappears. Sometimes with injured ligaments and tendons in the occipital region, say after a whiplash injury, one can experience an ache which mimics a headache. Massage the area affected or sore areas in the back of the head with balm or oil and the pain will disappear.

Headaches in the crown of the head are often due to increased fluid pressure in the brain. There could be a variety of reasons, from meningitis to tumours. Please consult a doctor immediately. In fact, if the headaches do not disappear after the treatments mentioned in this section you must consult a doctor for scans and a diagnosis.

If you have pain in the front of the head, especially when you try to read, then you need to have your eyesight checked. The eye muscles may be strained and you might require glasses or eye exercises to sort that out.

6.6 Ali Syndrome headaches

The most common form of headache is one-sided and with a neck problem on the corresponding side. If you suffer from frequent headaches, say more than once a week, which last up to a day and without sickness or photophobia (light sensitivity), then the chances are that some vertebrae on that side of the neck are misaligned. There could be a ligament or tendon injury in the area between the occiput at the back of the skull and the neck. Press these areas with your fingers and they will be painful. My massage-manipulative technique will help to eliminate such headaches.

The neck-type of headache is frequently associated with chronic fatigue, dizziness, muzzy head, palpitation and other symptoms of The Ali Syndrome.

In my opinion, migraine is like flu, or simple diarrhoea. It can heal on its own within 3 days. It is as if there is some imbalance in the body and when the balance is self-restored, the symptoms disappear. The migraine headache is very strong and has a devastating effect on both the mind and the body. People generally resort to strong painkillers, or anti-migraine drugs, which makes the blood less viscous so that it can flow with ease through the vessels to reach the brain tissue. Soon after taking these drugs, the pain disappears, but as the effect wears-off it runs with the same intensity. You need to repeat the intake of such drugs so that, after 3 days or so, it disappears completely on its own.

My main approach is to prepare the body in between attacks, so that the blood flow to the brain is uninterrupted and thus, when the attacks do come, the episode is mild or bearable, or there is a longer gap between them. In this case, it is important to have the treatment regularly for 3-4 months, when the headaches will finally go.

Summary: This description of the Ali Syndrome is probably best summed up by a description of actual cases I have treated using the technique.

Case Studies

My late friend, the film producer, Ismail Merchant (Howards' End, Room with a View), recommended me to an Arab gentleman, from a very respected family, because of his constant cluster headaches. This is a form of headache which happens once a year, especially in the spring to early summer period - more commonly in men. The headaches will be there daily, for a month or so, continuously. For the entire period the sufferer is debilitated and nothing except strong migraine pills and oxygen helps.

Anyway, the gentleman sent his plane to collect me from Stanstead Airport and I arrived at the destination late at night. Next morning, I saw him at 10am and he had an oxygen cylinder. The headaches were so severe that only oxygen helped him. No painkillers worked .I felt so sorry to see him with such pain. The very first question I asked was about any accident he had had. He was quite surprised, because he had had an accident when his four-wheel drive rolled over several times in the Arabian sand dunes, some four years prior to my visit. He immediately recalled that he had started getting headaches shortly after the accident. He hadn't linked the two and no doctor had asked him that question. He had seen specialists from various places, but none knew the cause of his headaches.

I touched his neck and it was extremely sore on the right side and so was the TMJ in front of the right jaw. He clenched his jaw whenever he had the pain from his headaches. He had not used the oxygen that morning and had a certain degree of pain. This pain went shortly after my initial treatment. That afternoon, he followed his passion and took his boat out to sea; dived for half an hour and fed the sharks.

I did visit him a few times and he had one of his therapists repeat the treatments daily. This treatment stopped the headaches. I had advised him to have regular treatments throughout the year. He had a spa area at his beach house and the therapists were from the Far East. This helped him to have less frequent headaches with less intensity. He did not need oxygen and life was comfortable. Cluster headaches are generally incurable but in this case he went into remission.

Angela, from the Midlands in UK, had headaches for 40 years, since childhood. She used to get headaches at least twice a week and lived on painkillers. She had read my column in The Mail on Sunday, where I answered the question from a headache sufferer and so she sought my advice as a last resort. I asked if she had dizziness, neck tension, fainting bouts as a teenager, along with nausea, irritability, lack of concentration, fatigue and sugar cravings. She answered 'yes' to all these symptoms. I then asked her if she had a birth injury and she immediately said that her mother had an almost 24 hours long and difficult labour and at the end forceps were used. She also had hurt her neck from some falls.

Angela came down to see me every week for four weeks and then twice a month for 3-4 months for treatment. That was the end of her headaches. She found a local sports massage therapist, whom she sees regularly. I have not seen her for almost ten years now. Menopause can cure the hormone-related monthly migraines, but frequent headaches like hers are cured only with increased blood supply to the brain.

* * * * *

A well-known chef in the UK used to get headaches every Saturday night at 11pm. He would return home early from his restaurant every Saturday as he expected the headache. He would get tightness in the neck, followed by a severe headache. He hated taking medicines for headaches but he saw no alternative. He would have headaches on Sundays and then feel absolutely fine by the evening. He had had allergy tests, but nothing showed any concrete evidence that they caused the headaches.

I put him on a diet that excluded yeast products, dairy, coffee, nuts, sugar, citrus fruits and alcohol. I saw him on Fridays. At first the intensity of headaches lessened and then he began not to have a headache on Saturdays. Today, he is free from headaches. I see him frequently on television and once, at a conference, I heard him talk about his headaches and he gave me credit for teaching him the right diet and for applying the exact treatment. The Ali technique of therapy helped him to be symptom-free.

6.7 Dizziness and Vertigo

Dizziness is a milder version of vertigo which is a condition with a tendency to whirling. You feel as if your surroundings are moving around you. If you turn round and round in one spot and suddenly stop, the world around you seems to move and you loose balance.

Dizziness, or giddiness, is becoming more common due to stress, computer use, driving, flying in aircrafts with uncomfortable headrests, changing pillows due to frequent travelling etc. With the slightest movement of the head one experiences these symptoms.

Vertigo is a violent attack of extreme dizziness. The eyes roll and you lose total balance and collapse on the floor, unless you hold onto something to prevent it from happening. You get very panicky and the heart races. Sometimes, you feel as if you are going to pass out. I have experienced it once myself.

* * * * *

In 1988, I went on an Indian Ocean Island called Lakshwadeep, close to the Maldives with the Indian Presidential Party. I was treating the First Lady for a condition. A special village was built with pre-fabricated houses and I had one right on the beach. The President, with his officials, went about their engagements. I asked the Naval officers, who were there for security reasons, if they could take me snorkelling.

A high-speed rubber dingy arrived and took me to an area with pristine coral reefs. I put on the glasses and the tube and jumped into the sea. What I saw was paradise. A big fish swam past me. The corals and sea world, with numerous varieties of fish was so beautiful. I was totally engrossed in that world. As I was warned that there were sharks in these waters, I was on the lookout. When I bent my neck to look ahead, my eyes went dark and my limbs were numb. Then, suddenly, I felt the sea churning around me. The Naval Officer saw me going limp and jumped into the water. We were all in our skin suits. He pulled me onto the boat. The vertigo was very scary. I thought I was going to die.. As the boat rocked, it felt worse but with some presence of mind, I began to squeeze my neck with my hands. Somehow, I managed to tell them to lie me flat with my head right down and to massage my neck and shoulder. Once horizontal, I felt slightly better, but very nervous. The Naval Officer panicked and started the boat to take me back to the shore. I think he tried to radio the medical post, but I told them what it was and they calmed down. My neck was very sore and the jumpy movements of the small boat over the waves made the situation worse.

They took the boat right up to my unit; I staggered across the beach and peeled my clothes off. I lay on my back and asked the Naval Officer to give my neck a pull. They were so kind and did what I asked of them. If I hadn't been a doctor, I am sure I would have landed-up in the Medical Inspection Room. After only a few minutes, I felt calmer. I continued to breathe very slowly, holding my breath for up to 15 seconds and my heart rate came down. I felt extremely sleepy. I lay on the floor and asked the officers to leave after thanking them for their help.

I had been busy on that Presidential Tour. We went to Cochin from Delhi and spent the night there, flew in helicopters to a naval ship, had lunch with the entire crew, slept in cabins with a strong smell of diesel; saw naval exercises on high seas with aircraft, mock fights, helicopter rescues, sonar detection of submarines etc. It was great fun watching the exercises with The President and his family, but it was no doubt very exhausting, especially as I had to do treatments as well. I hardly slept at night because of uncomfortable beds and different environments.

All that tightened my neck and the sudden movement of the head must have misaligned a vertebra in my neck, causing an acute reduction in blood flow to my brain. Fortunately, I knew what it was and organised my own treatment. I was well by the evening and attended a folk dance performance on the makeshift helipad. The news of my illness was revealed to the Presidential Party and they were all very concerned. I felt embarrassed, as I was the doctor. That evening in the officer's mess where the senior officers dined, we had a good laugh. Later that evening, when I went to see the First Lady, she asked me what had happened. News does spread fast.

* * * * *

The secretary of an important Arab dignitary and businessman in the Middle East, worked long hours on computers. He suffered from insomnia and had had an unhealthy lifestyle for several years at a stretch. It started off as fatigue, headaches, slight dizziness, blurred vision and short-term memory loss. As time went by, he began to get palpitations. One day, while driving on the main highway, he had an extreme attack of vertigo. He swerved the car sideways onto the grass verge, flung open the door and lay flat on the ground. He began to shake violently, as if he was having an epileptic fit. Some people gathered round and took him to hospital.

After a lot of investigations, including brain scans, nothing substantial showed-up. He was put on a tablet for vertigo and it was diagnosed as an inner ear problem. This is the most common diagnosis for extreme dizziness and vertigo. I was in the country on a routine visit. I examined him and my diagnosis was the lack of blood flow to the cerebellum, due to extreme tightness of the neck muscles. His boss half-believed my diagnosis and gave me the benefit of the doubt. As requested, he joined me with a group of patients on one of my health trips to a remote castle in Rajasthan.

He responded positively to treatment and he felt very relaxed and energetic. One day we had to take a 3 hour bus journey on a bumpy road. He fell asleep on the bus and had his neck in an awkward position. When we reached the castle, he tried to get up but had another attack of vertigo. His eyes moved rapidly, as if following the whirling of the world around him and he was almost unconscious. He then had a mild seizure. I had just got off the bus when this happened. I went back and had him lie on his back in the passageway and immediately began to work on his neck. I gave it a bit of traction with my hands. As soon as he felt a bit better he tried to get up but had another attack of vertigo. He panicked, as do the majority of people in this situation. It is very scary, as you feel you are going to die.

There wasn't a stretcher, as it is a remote castle. I used a blanket and, with the help of a few people, carried him to his room- the round gun room – where, 300 years ago, stood the main cannon that defended against the invading enemies from the East. We had the maestro, Sultan Khan, a very well known musician, who played an ancient instrument called the Sarangi, a stringed instrument which is played with a bow and very similar to a small Cello. Without any hesitation, he sat in the centre of this large, round room with a dome and began to play a tune. The sound of the Sarangi is very similar to the human singing voice. As my patient lay flat on his back, without a pillow, I gave him some water to drink, with the help of a tablespoon, as he could not lift his head, lest it triggered another attack.

I gently treated his neck and felt the misalignment of the neck vertebrae. Sultan Khan's music was divine as it echoed in the domed room. I have never treated anyone in such superb ambiance. I was totally enchanted by the music of one of the geniuses of Indian music. My patient drifted-off into a deep state of relaxation. About half an hour later, he got-up to use the toilet. It was miraculous. The notes of the Sarangi had enhanced the therapeutic effect of my treatment a thousand times.

Next morning he was in the courtyard talking to a few people in the group who were enquiring how he felt. He was calm and relaxed, joking with everyone. It was impossible to imagine the situation he was in the previous evening. His treatment continued and he is now totally cured. I met him seven years later; he had taken a couple of years off to study, but he had returned to his job. He never had another vertigo attack again.

* * * * *

A dear friend of mine, Silas Chou, whom I have known for over twenty-five years, owned a very successful garment business. Some of the labels are, like Tommy Hilfiger and Michael Kors, world famous. One morning, after his routine jogging, he felt extreme vertigo and collapsed on the floor. His wife called me immediately and I contacted Dr Nachi, a friend at The Harley Street Clinic and he kindly rushed to Chester Square, where Silas lived. He was admitted to The Charing Cross Hospital. He was diagnosed with an inner ear problem. I knew it was his neck that was responsible for the vertigo attack. He flew regularly to New York and Hong Kong on his private jet. We used to say that he lived on his plane and he only landed, from time to time, to stretch his legs.

I went to the hospital and his face looked pale. He was on medication and his darling wife Celia looked very concerned. I explained how neck stiffness can restrict blood flow to the brain, sometimes acutely after some violent movement (in his case after jogging). They knew about my theory and no convincing was necessary. I massaged his neck, which was extremely sore to touch. When he felt better, another mild episode started when he tried to get-up to go to the toilet. I made him lie flat on his back and continued treatment for over 2 hours until he fell asleep.

CT scans of the brain and inner ear were taken and some other tests, which involved water and a tilted bed, were carried out. There was some grit, or crystals, found in the ear. In this case, there was a problem with the ear as well as the neck condition. He was discharged from hospital and I gave him more treatments at home. He began to fly again. He also had some more tests in America and the inner ear disease called Meniere's Disease was diagnosed. I told him to have regular neck massages and exercises. He travels much less now and has not had any more attacks .As friends we meet each other from time to time , even though he lives in New York.

My question is that if crystals in the inner ear caused it, why was it so acute and only happened for one short period of a few days? I agree that Stugeron or Stemetil are drugs that suppress car sickness, dizziness and vertigo, but they don't actually cure them. Silas changed his lifestyle; had regular neck and shoulder massages, as instructed, and does regular exercises. He is now cured.

Elderly people suffer frequently from imbalance. They feel that the floor is swaying as if in an earthquake. They begin to walk awkwardly, fixing their eyes on the surface on which they walk. This changes their posture and they often develop a 'hunch back'. They often shuffle their feet and that is sometimes mistaken as Parkinsonism. A former Prime Minister of a big country walked very slowly and shuffled his feet. Tests showed he had a degenerative knee joint. Everyone thought he couldn't walk because of his knee. A top surgeon from the US was called in and his knee was replaced. His walking did not improve, even after many months of physiotherapy. I was invited to see him. At first glance, I could tell he had imbalance. Moving his head from left to right a few times caused dizziness. I made him stand, close his eyes and told him to walk. He lost his balance and nearly fell down.

I discussed his imbalance with his doctor, a leading orthopaedic surgeon. He didn't believe me. I asked the patient about accidents. He quietly told me that as a teenager he wrestled a lot and was dropped on his neck and shoulder numerous time in the sand.

I suggested treatment under my care but because of security issues he couldn't travel much. What followed later was heartbreaking. The advanced complications of neck connection followed. After a few years he had a stroke and was bed ridden. He has lost memory and has signs of dementia. It is very sad because he was a very bright man, a writer and a poet. He is a well-respected politician of this populous democracy.

Motion Sickness

This is an extremely unpleasant sensation and includes dizziness, headaches, sweating, flushing of the face, nausea, vomiting and mood alterations. At first, sufferers may feel the excitement of giddiness with palpitation, but then they have extreme disgust and can even feel suicidal. It happens when the body (head) moves in a car or on a ship that rocks or tilts from side to side in the sea. In rough seas almost everyone gets these symptoms.

The inner ear has a unique device to detect this type of body movement. There are 3 semi-circular tubes that are positioned horizontally, vertically and front to back. These canals have fluids, so if you move your head from left to right, or vice versa, the horizontal semicircular canal picks-up this motion and sends impulses through the nerves to the middle brain. A similar situation arises when you bend your head forward and backwards and when you move up and down. They cover all three major aspects of the body movement and their permutations and combinations. This part of the inner ear, which deals with equilibrium is called the vestibule (passageway). The adjacent part of the inner ear is called the cochlear (shell which resembles a snail's back). This apparatus picks-up sound. We will deal with this part under 'Tinnitus'.

The vestibule and the cochlear are embedded near the ear, in the section of the temporal bone. They are extremely well protected, as there are delicate membranes which have highly sensitive nerve endings, responsible for equilibrium, balance and hearing. There are two separate nerves; the vestibular is responsible for equilibrium and the cochlear is responsible for hearing and they join together to form the Vestibular-cochlear nerve. This is a thick nerve that ends-up in the midbrain, from where the vestibular impulses send messages to the cerebellum (the rear brain) for assessment and control of both balance and postural adjustments. Motion sickness is probably due to a failure of the cerebellum to cope with too frequent and too rapid changes in posture. Balance control is a slow process as too many muscles need to be re-adjusted at the same time.

The eyes, too, play a part in balance control. They fathom the height of the head from the ground and the distances of objects around you in order to adjust your posture, so that you don't fall. So when you rotate your body in one place, or go on a merry-go-round, your balance is upset for a few minutes after stopping. The eyes see objects go round in quick succession. When you stand on a wall to jump down, you are scared because your body's height is added to the height of the wall and therefore, you feel much higher than you actually are. It is a greater height than you could actually jump from and you then sit on the wall to reduce the total height and jump.

For sea-sickness, which is a part of motion sickness, sailors will tell you to look at the horizon and fix your eyes there and not on the sea, which is tilting sideways all the time. Fixing the eyes also stabilizes the neck . This reduces the risk of vertebral arteries compression due to lateral movement of the neck.. Some patients, who go with me to the Himalayas for my health programme, get car sickness due to the winding roads. The car constantly turns to the left and then to the right and the road to Shimla has notorious turns and bends, as it was built for slow moving cars and horse carriages. The British went up to the hills from Delhi for almost nine months a year to beat the heat of the plains. It was the summer capital of India. Today's fast cars make the journey very unpleasant and people prefer the small train journey.

I have noticed that on my Himalayan trips to higher altitudes, the neck massage and manipulation helps people to cope much better with both motion and altitude sickness. For example, in the beginning motion sickness in some people would be horrendous. I advise them to fix their eyes on a distant point on the road and not to look out of the window. This is difficult, as the scenery is spectacular. Some close their eyes and sleep. This helps. After a few days, with regular treatments, which all patients have, the motion sickness improves. If you have smaller meals the vomiting then reduces, but the nausea remains the same. I give the vulnerable people anti-sickness pills and even antihistamines with strong sedative properties. This knocks them out for a while and when they wake-up, they don't panic and the journey becomes much easier. In the early days, when we used a bus for our Himalayan journey, my staff would give the guests neck massages every hour or so. This would tremendously help those who were susceptible to fatigue, muzzy head and car sickness .

* * * * *

A lady in her seventies began to get a phobia of getting into a car. Every time the car accelerated or braked, she felt nauseous. She lived in central London, where the traffic is erratic; it made her movements within town almost impossible. I had treated her for headaches and dizziness already. I was aware of her chronic constipation, which caused poor calcium absorption, as this element, along with magnesium, are predominantly absorbed in the colon. She later had osteoporosis due to calcium deficiency, as a result of which the neck shrank a little. This caused her circulatory problems. I treated her constipation, gave high quality coral calcium in water, massaged her neck regularly and gave her some exercises. After a few sessions, her symptoms disappeared. She had spent a lot of time and money investigating the problem, even though the solution was simple.

6.8 Tinnitus

Tinnitus is the hearing of noises where there is no sound in the surrounding environment. This noise could be buzzing (bee, mosquito or bumble-bee sounds), ringing (a constant ringing of a bell), a steam engine or pulsating sound, corresponding to the heart rate or pulse, a high pitched noise or whistling and all the variations of these sounds. A loud bang or noise at rock concerts and discotheques can kick-start tinnitus. In this case the noise 'damages' the sensitive hearing nerve endings in the cochlear-part of the inner ear.

* * * * *

A friend of mine was in a building in New Delhi which collapsed after a large explosion. He was buried under the rubble for three hours. He was with his girlfriend, who sadly died. He had a lot of damage to the neck vertebrae, a couple of which had to be surgically fused. For years now he has suffered from severe headaches, dizziness, nausea, tinnitus, deafness, anxiety, insomnia, chronic fatigue etc; in fact, full blown Ali Syndrome. Most of the symptoms went away with my treatment, but tinnitus and deafness remains. He is used to it now.

* * * * *

I must confess, unless someone with tinnitus comes to me within 6 months of its onset, I cannot do much to eliminate it. When I treat tinnitus using my techniques, especially in the early days, the sound disappears soon after the session. They can bring it on simply by thinking about it. I always tell them to keep the 'sound' out of their mind, once it disappears after the treatment sessions. This part is extremely difficult because some people get very agitated with the constant ringing or buzzing. It is said that Van Gogh had tinnitus and the sound irritated him so much that he cut off his ear. Meditation, deep breathing and sound sleep helps to push the thought of the sound into the background. The treatment helps to diminish the sound, but one has to use will power to keep that away. It's better not to remind oneself of the sound altogether.

I sometimes recommend Ginko Biloba and B-Complex, in addition to the neck treatment, in order to facilitate recovery in the early stages of the disease. The neck treatment should be done professionally once a week for 8 weeks or so, but the patient should also self massage the neck, the jaw on the affected side and the area below the base of the ear. This area is extremely sore in people with tinnitus. Massage gently for 3-4 minutes and then deeply for another 4 minutes. It's best when someone else does the treatment, especially when everything is so sensitive to touch.

Sometimes blocked ears, due to a closed Eustachian Tube, can exacerbate the symptoms. In that case, put 2 drops of my Sinus Oil, or sesame oil, into the nostrils and sniff. After a couple of minutes, try to 'pop' the ears, as you would in an aeroplane. For some this 'pop' will not happen immediately and so you have to try, morning and evening, for several days until the tube that connects the throat to the middle ear (the Eustachian Tube) opens-up.

Almost immediately after 'popping', the hearing improves. So, if one suffers from slight hearing loss (which is not caused by nerve damage, an explosion or punctured ear drum) as well as tinnitus, which is often the case, the hearing- loss cannot mask tinnitus but can be pushed to the background. You need to keep the sinus decongested and the Eustachian tubes clear by avoiding cheese, ice cream, chilled drinks, cream, yoghurt and excess sugar. Also, make sure the bowels move regularly, by drinking more water (at least 6-8 glasses per day); eat figs, papaya, prunes, spinach, beetroot etc, as chronic constipation causes the sinuses to become congested due to a toxic mucous discharge.

Tinnitus is difficult to cure because there is a lot a patient needs to do. A therapist, or Integrated Physician, may do the treatment using my technique, but the patient has to participate in his or her own treatment by following the diet, keeping the Eustachian tubes clear, doing self massage, sleeping well and staying calm. The ball is really in their court and only the disciplined succeed in overcoming it. The entire therapy is done as a complex; just massage alone may not be enough.

Conventional medical treatment is limited to using a special hearing aid that produces a more acceptable sound to mask the unpleasant and irritating noises. Acupuncture has been successful in a limited number of cases.

In my opinion, the auditory nerve, which comprises the vestibular (for balance) and the cochlear (for hearing), is a thick nerve. It is fed by branches of the vertebro-basilar artery. Tinnitus, especially that which is not caused by sound damage, responds better with improved blood supply through these arteries. This is limited to the ringing or whistling type of tinnitus. After disembarking from a long-haul flight, one often has fatigue, a muzzy head, along with mild tinnitus. Perhaps this is from constant engine noise over a period of time. A good therapeutic massage after the flight and ample rest and rehydration, eliminates tinnitus quickly. Sometimes those who live in noisy urban areas experience tinnitus when they go to the countryside for the weekend or holiday, which is much quieter. There is a residual noise in the ears for a couple of days. Once rested, the noise disappears. A major artery to the brain passes very close to the hearing apparatus of the cochlear in the inner ear. Plaque deposits in the artery may cause turbulence and noise from the flow of blood in the artery. This sound, which corresponds to the heartbeat or pulse, has a periodic 'whooshing' tone. This type of tinnitus does not respond to neck treatments as the cause is different.

Some people hear a fairly constant 'popping' sound. This is usually due to the partially blocked Eustachian tube letting in air into the middle ear. As I mentioned, this tube originates in the upper part of the throat and ends in the middle ear. Its main purpose is to blow the walls of the middle ear to form a chamber, in which three tiny bones are located. One lies behind the ear drum and the other lies in front of the window of the inner ear, which picks-up the vibration and transfers it to the nerve endings. The middle bone connects these two other bones. These bones simply transfer the vibrations of the ear drum to where they can be converted into electrical nerve impulses, which are taken to the brain via the auditory nerve to be interpreted as sound.

When the Eustachian tube is blocked, due to a throat or middle ear infection, the air bubbles disappear and the bones cannot be suspended in 'midair' to vibrate efficiently. This leads to hearing loss.

* * * * *

The owner of a garment chain had tinnitus a few months after a car accident. It disturbed him very much, as it was high-pitched and continuous. Someone recommended him to see me. He said he would do anything to get rid of it. I gave him frequent treatments, as it was a complaint which was still only a few weeks old. He did the yoga exercises; followed a diet with no excess salt, sugar and coffee to calm down the nerves. It worked quite quickly. His tinnitus disappeared, only to return after a long-haul flight. He came back to me immediately and it was resolved again. After a few episodes, it stopped. He understood the trigger and began to manage it well.

My advice is that Tinnitus can become chronic. It rarely goes without treatment and it is an annoying condition, especially when you focus on it all the time. Stay calm and ask someone to massage your neck before you seek professional help from a trained therapist. Check the treatment method described later in this book.

6.9 Nausea and Sickness

If you are anaemic, the oxygen supply to the brain is restricted due to lack of Haemoglobin. This causes fatigue, slight nausea and breathlessness on exertion. All these symptoms get worse when you smell wet paint, petrol fumes or walk into a crowded place or smoky environment. The oxygen in the air is reduced in these conditions and so you feel very nauseous or sick; sickness is a result of extreme nausea.

Similarly, when the neck restricts blood supply to the subconscious brain, nausea or sickness are common symptoms, especially when you move. If the oxygen level is low in the environment, the nausea materialises into vomiting. During my high altitude journeys across the Himalayas with groups of patients, nausea, sickness and vomiting were common symptoms. I then introduced neck massages during acclimatization below 9000 feet (2800 metres) and the participants of my Himalayan programmes no longer suffered these problems. In 1994, everybody, including myself, had severe nausea at 11000 feet. Every year since then, I have had to spend more time in Manali (7000 feet) to acclimatize. Then in 2003, I took my therapists along and we needed just 3 days of acclimatization at 9000 feet. After the treatments, all the 12 participants, including one who had had part of her lung removed due to cancer, crossed the 16,500 feet Bhaba Pass without a hitch. For the first time, all of us had the breathlessness, but no sickness. The only variable was the special neck treatment. After that, I included this treatment on every trip and no one has had any problems with the altitude since.

Basically, with lack of oxygen supply one gets nausea. Sickness is the body's own way of elimination of fluids from the gut. As a result of that, the body gets dehydrated and the blood becomes 'thicker'. There is more haemoglobin per ml of blood, so more oxygen can be absorbed. Temporarily, this fixes the problem of oxygen supply to the brain; thicker blood means more oxygen concentration.

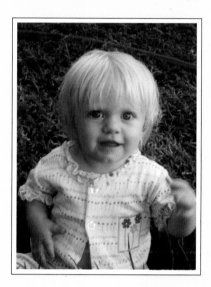

I was visiting my friends Gaynor and Johann Rupert in South Africa for Christmas and New Year. On Christmas Day, I saw a little girl Chloe of nine months who was brought to me. Chloe was the daughter of their Farm Manager in the Karoo. She looked pale and her hands and feet were cold. The parents drove down for several hours to see me and were very worried. She had a tiny feeding tube in her stomach. For six months she had projectile vomiting after every feed. She could not retain anything. She had a few operations and was fed upside down to let the food go up the stomach. They were told she had multiple food intolerances and there was nothing concrete could be done. She also suffered from frequent bladder infection, was nauseous along with gagging and retching. She was tired and slept a lot as a result of chronic fatigue. The doctor finally thought she was 'neurotic'. They prescribed antidepressant.

I asked her parents about her birth. She was a caesarean baby. I then asked if there had been a fall or accident. At first they couldn't recall any trauma. My brain ticked to find the right clue. I touched her neck and she was visibly uncomfortable. I started massaging the neck and her parents were getting concerned as their baby began to cry. Suddenly her mother recalled the trauma. When she was three months old and lying in bed, her elder sister jumped on her and she had cried a lot. The nausea and vomiting started shortly after that. There was a direct, definite link between the trauma and symptoms.

I then explained what had happened. The trauma had affected her neck and so she had problems with blood flow to the brain. This had caused the fatigue, nausea, retching and a poor immune system (hence the frequent bladder infections). It sounded like Greek to them, but they gave me a chance. After fifteen minutes of treatment of the neck, jaw, throat, scalp, shoulders and upper back, her face turned pink and her cheeks were red. I said that was because the blood was flowing into the head. This convinced the parents of my diagnosis, as she had always been so pale.

Next morning, they came to see me. Her mother was very excited as the baby had drunk 50 mls of milk for the first time without vomiting. They always thought she was allergic to milk. She had been on formula milk since she was only three days old. That was a big relief, as I needed the parents' faith and cooperation. I wanted them to massage her neck 2-3 times a day.

I taught them the technique and massaged the mother's neck to demonstrate the appropriate pressure and technique.

I saw the baby for a week. Everyday there was something new to report. They kept in touch with me via email and sent me photos of her progress. She has grown to be a delightful child; active, chatty and even a little mischievous. The feeding tube was removed and she now eats everything. I expect her to grow up to be a tall girl. As I will explain later, by stimulating the Pituitary gland with a proper blood supply, the Growth Hormone secretion normally increases which boosts a growth spurt.

* * * * *

A lady from a highly respected family in the UK had suffered from sickness for over nine months. She had lost almost three stones in weight. Every possible test had been done, but nothing substantially wrong could be found. Her family was extremely worried. The doctors had diagnosed it as a psychological problem.

She had been given all sorts of tablets. After every meal she would be sick and sometimes even drinking water would produce the same result.

Initially, the doctors looked for stomach ulcers and then viral gastric flu. They desperately tried to find a proper cause or diagnoses. Sadly, a lot of drugs had been prescribed which not only suppressed the appetite, but also made her zombie-like, which was picked-up as depression. The weight loss did not help, as she became very tired and malnourished. She would eat small meals, 6-10 a day, and sometimes she could retain a little of that food. That sustained her basic energy.

I was asked to go and see her. She lived alone in the country, but her daughter had come down to assist with all the further arrangements.

I examined her tongue and she looked dehydrated. Some vertebrae in the neck were misaligned. I asked her to move her head sideways for five times and that caused dizziness. All the telltale signs of the neck connection were there.

Then I asked her about an accident. She said she had none. I gave her some clues, and when I asked if she slipped on the pavement and fell. She recalled immediately that three years previously, she had fallen very badly in her house. The carpet near the stairs did not have any grip and she slipped on the wooden floor. She had hit the back of her head and suffered from concussion. Afterwards, she had some headaches and dizziness.

I explained what had happened. She couldn't understand the link, but wanted to give the treatment a try. After the first couple of treatments, she responded well and her appetite returned. I told her to eat soft nutritious foods. She ate pureed vegetables, mashed potatoes, mushy rice, minced meat, grilled or steamed fish, fresh juices, cottage cheese, porridge etc. She avoided citric juices, so that there would be no gastric irritation.

She felt more energetic and began to walk in fresh air. Her sickness stopped. I would have loved to have continued the treatment, but she lived in the country and could not come down to London to see me and it was not possible for me to drive down every week to see her. Unfortunately we lost touch, but I presume she is better.

6.10 The Emotional Element

I was always fascinated by Psychiatry as a subject. Even when I was about twelve, I used to go to the American Library in Calcutta, during my holidays from my boarding school, to read books on this subject. In the final year of my MD course in Moscow, I used to spend my free time and do night duties in Hospital No 8, a Psychiatric Institute. I was very interested in Anorexia Nervosa, which was beginning to spread amongst young women in the former Soviet Union. I did a paper for the Student's Scientific Society, almost like a mini-thesis, comparing the condition with a mild form of Schizophrenia. Critics will now disagree, but in those days it was well accepted.

As I mentioned earlier, when blood flow is reduced to the brain, people can get various psychological and emotional problems. A slight reduction of blood flow tends to produce symptoms like fatigue, drowsiness, lethargy, depression, sighing, "sinking feeling in the head.", lack of motivation, lack of concentration, feeling "detached" (as if watching a TV film where you are not participating), zombie feeling, fear. A more moderate decrease in blood flow will produce anxiety, panic attacks, irritability, lack of reasoning, excessive talking, phobias (in chronic condition), being excessively suspicious, obsessiveness, hyperactivity, "high-pitched" voice, severe insomnia. Severe restriction of blood can cause severe panic attacks, tremor with rage, fainting and other more pronounced reactions.

The above symptoms are subjective and cannot be measured unless on a scale of 1 to 10 to assess the severity. They are generally treated under "psychological and emotional" problems. Antidepressants, tranquillisers, sedatives are generally used to "mask" the symptoms so that people can carry on with their lives without affecting the people around them with their unreasonable behaviour.

I must clarify that depression is a very common symptom prevalent in society. There are two types of this condition. The first is a symptom of the Ali Syndrome where lack of blood flow is the primary cause. You reinstate the blood flow and the symptoms are reversed. The other more serious condition is Clinical Depression which is an organic disease. Here, the disease is deep-rooted. The lack of neurochemicals, like serotonin, is a noticeable marker of this disease. Unless these chemicals are replaced, the Depression as a disease cannot be easily cured. Similarly, if lack of insulin gives Type I diabetes, it is essential to inject the hormone to keep the blood sugar in check. Hormone replacement therapy is essential for Thyroid malfunction, as for Ovarian, Testicular, or Adrenal malfunctions.

In Clinical Depression, the symptoms are more pronounced. People cry, have morbid thought, even of suicide, a feeling of listlessness and total lack of motivation or decision-making capacity. Such patients can't work and are stubborn in their thoughts. There is no way my neck treatment will cure that without supportive therapies (drugs, meditation, change of environment, psychotherapy etc).

A young lady came to see me with full-blown Ali Syndrome symptoms. She had chronic fatigue, dull headache, jet lag-type sleep disturbances, (tired during the day, awake at night), lack of concentration, dizziness, hormonal imbalance (severe acne, in her 30s, facial hair, dark pigmentation on the skin, low thyroid function), craving for sugar, palpitations, hyperventilation, blurred vision, occasional tinnitus, intolerance to wet paint or petrol fumes etc. Additionally, she had severe panic attacks, restless leg syndrome (tossing and turning), vivid dreams (almost awake), in her sleep - screaming, sleep-walking, bruxism (grinding of teeth); multiple phobia (flying, insects, dirty toilets, claustrophobia). She also had a feeling of being pregnant, even when she was in her safe period, frequent mood swings, severe premenstrual syndrome, lasting for two weeks before the periods. She couldn't work as she hated everything in the office. She felt suffocated and hated her colleagues. Additionally, she had Crohn's disease (an autoimmune disorder). I asked her if she had any injuries. She couldn't recall any. I gave her hints like car or motorbike accidents, falls, excessive dental work, knock on the head, swimming pool accidents etc. She couldn't recall any such traumas to the head and neck. When I asked her about being hit on the head by someone, she broke down and it took a large part of the allocated consultation time to calm her down. In childhood she was beaten very badly by her mother, who once tried to strangle her. She was slapped and her head was banged against the wall on several occasions. Then her boyfriend was violent as well. I could clearly see the picture.

I wrote down everything, as she had severe short-term memory loss. I showed her the model of the neck and a section of the brain and explained her limbic system (responsible for emotions, sleep, motivation, drive), the Pituitary-hypothalamic area (responsible for the hormonal imbalance, palpitations, Crohn's Disease etc), and other parts of the subconscious brain were malfunctioning due to the neck problem and subsequent lack of blood flow. She immediately complained of extreme neck tension and constant discomfort. She had dizziness when I asked her to move her head to the left and right.

A couple of days later, I gave her a neck treatment and gently manipulated it. She had instant rush of blood to the head. She flushed and said that the room looked brighter. She began to cry. She later said the quality of sleep had improved, but she felt like crying all the time (depression).

After a few treatments, she felt a lot better. She opened up and began to tell me more about her personal life. She started yoga, changed her diet and had weekly neck treatments. Today she is a transformed woman. Her skin, her energy, her moods, her digestion and her outlook towards life have improved dramatically.

* * * * *

I often wondered if my treatment would influence drug and alcohol addiction. I took several cases of cocaine, marijuana, alcohol and social drug addiction. I would take care not to do anything that would cause "cold turkey" in the withdrawal phase. A young woman with a successful career was addicted to cocaine. She was instructed to give up cocaine. She received a daily 2-hour neck and body massage. The drug seemed to have settled in the muscles and liver because of the smaller blood vessels. She drank soup and fresh vegetable juice, water, herbal tea and my Detox Tea. As expected, she felt very drowsy and slept for up to 16 hours a day in the first few days. Cocaine makes you "awake" so its withdrawal causes drowsiness. After a week, she felt a lot better.

I sent her to the Himalayas to the place where I usually treat chronic patients. She had two hours of massage, did yoga and walked in the mountains every day. Some of the walks were tough, and she complained. My assistant encouraged and motivated her to walk further. Every time she would climb atop a hill, she was encouraged to say. "I can do it; it's not difficult for me anymore". This gave her the positive affirmation. The feel-good factor created by the neck treatment played a very positive role. She is now off drugs, with a good chance, forever.

* * * * *

In alcohol addiction too, similar treatments can help a lot. The diet/juices help the liver to detox. Neck massage creates the energy and feel-good factor and walking in the mountains, helps to build willpower. With a determined effort, supported by a boost in energy, addicts are able to quit their habits.

I would like my treatment to be used to help with addictions and emotional problems. It is an area crying out for research by the many organisations already involved in these cases.

6.11 Eating Disorders

When I moved to London from Hong Kong, I became aware that eating disorders were quite common the UK. Bulimia and binging were quite widespread. Those who suffer from this condition, feel quite 'full' after eating. As they eat fast and excessively, they feel tired and even slightly nauseous. It is because if this feeling, some make themselves sick to relieve the feeling. The nausea, in some women, is definitely a trigger point. I began to think about these women. The ritual of forced vomiting then becomes conditioned and they do it after every major meal.

I came up with the idea of my neck treatment to stop the nausea after meals. After a heavy meal, the blood rushes to the abdomen to aid digestion (the secretion of juices, the churning of food, the movement of digested matter further down the GI tract), which is a taxing mechanical process. When that happens, the brain is deprived of blood. If one has severe neck problems, the blood flow to the brain is reduced even further, so the nausea becomes more prominent.

* * * * *

The daughter of a successful Asian business man from Bombay went to boarding school in England. She missed home and she developed some depression. When she was sixteen years old, she became bulimic. In Asian families this sort of condition is alarming as daughters do have to get married. Bulimia, a psychological condition, is a no-no for a match to a suitable boy and they get rejected by the groom's family. She couldn't tell anyone, not even her parents and siblings, as she feared the worst. How she managed to hide it from her family during the holidays is a miracle.

She approached me. I began to give her neck massages, taught her yoga, gave her some herbal antacids and gave her some tips on relaxation. I also told her to lie down flat, without a pillow, soon after a meal so that the blood could flow to her brain with more ease. This integrated approach began to help. Her nausea after meals reduced and then disappeared. She usually fell asleep after meals. When she woke-up after a nap, she didn't feel the need to be sick. That was my first case of bulimia and my system worked. Today she is married and has children.

* * * * *

A couple of years ago a beautiful lady, in her mid-forties came to see me with fatigue and insomnia. She had had several horse-riding and skiing accidents and also suffered with headaches, nausea and palpitations. I suggested she went on my Himalayan Programme for treatment for Chronic Fatigue Syndrome. She made child-care arrangements and booked onto the trip.

In the Himalayas, I noticed she was very fidgety. She would eat quite a lot and walk about in the dining room feeling quite restless. After a week, I asked her why she looked so disturbed and restless at times. She then told me the real story.

As a teenager, she was anorexic but was cured. Some ten years later, she had a lot of stress and she became bulimic. She suffered for fifteen years and her nausea and urge to be sick reduced in the Himalayas, but her stomach automatically went into spasm. Even the abdominal muscles contracted after meals, as if she was retching. This was a disturbing feeling, which she did not want to experience, and it was for this reason she was so restless. She started to attend the meditation classes in the evening. The neck massage, yoga and meditation gave her the strength to overcome a long battle with bulimia. She now feels how silly the whole thing was. You eat and then make yourself sick? What a nuisance the entire thing was!

* * * * *

Perhaps not all bulimics can be treated in this way. Some are seriously psychologically motivated and those women need help. I have only a dozen cases where I was successful in eliminating the problem. There were some, especially with binging, who lost patience after a couple of sessions. They need a quick-fix, like a drug, that will help immediately, so that they can gain confidence.

Cravings for Sugar as Food

The appetite centre is located in the Hypothalamus. It tells us when we are hungry so that we get the drive to procure food and we then go out to purchase food or start cooking something to eat at home. It also tells us when we are full so that we can stop eating. The feeling of satiety is also obtained from the stomach muscles being stretched to their maximum capacity. If the glucose levels in the blood drop, the Hypothalamus gets panicky,

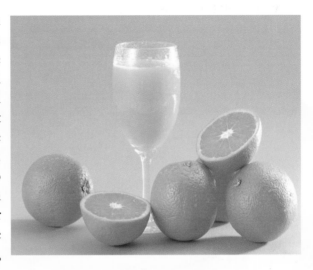

as the brain needs fuel all the time. It creates an appetite, or hunger, and drives us to find food. Simultaneously, one gets irritated and some even get headaches with hunger. If neck problems restrict blood flow to the Hypothalamus, it begins to react in a similar way, as the amount of glucose it receives is low around meal times. When the stomach is empty the accumulation of acid in it irritates the nerve endings on its walls, which then creates hunger pangs. The more acid you have the more you want to eat. So, on an empty stomach, in people with neck problems, food cravings are very strong. If you don't see food on the plate you get very upset. Thus the expression 'a hungry man is an angry man'.

A craving for sugar, or sweets, is more prominent with stress, excessive computer use, insomnia, lengthy drives etc. The neck muscles tighten and get an instant craving for glucose. After a meal, when blood rushes to the abdomen, the glucose supply to the Appetite Centre in the Hypothalamus is reduced. Additionally, if you have a neck condition, the cravings become unbearable. Many people crave for something sweet a few minutes after a meal. That is why desserts are served at the end of a meal. Sugar suppresses the craving immediately.

When one gets cravings for sugar or one is very hungry, a small amount of sugar can suppress the craving and you don't need an entire chocolate bar to achieve this! What happens is that the sweet-tasting buds on the tongue pick-up the signal and send it to the Hypothalamus, which then sends the message to the liver to release stored glucose. The sugar (sucrose) one eats cannot be digested immediately, as it takes a while to be split into glucose by amylase in the saliva or pancreatic juice. Glucose is the only form of sugar that is found in the blood and can be transported into the cells. Therefore, the sugar one eats acts via the taste buds.

You can use this phenomenon to temporarily stop your food cravings. Take a polo mint, or a couple of raisins and you will feel the cravings subside as soon as you put them into your mouth. The liver stores glycogen: a complex form of glucose.

Food, especially sugar cravings, is one of the many causes of weight gain. Those who have problems with binging have the worst form of psychologically-induced cravings. They will secretly buy, or store chocolates, fruit bars, sweets etc. Some cannot resist sweet shops. The traders, too, prey on such people. They display a variety of chocolates, sweets, bars etc of all different brands. Even though the main ingredient is sugar, cocoa, butter etc the chemical flavourings alter the taste to cater to the individual's needs. It is just like the different brands of cigarettes on display,

In my weight loss plan, which I am using in the Castel Monastero Spa in Tuscany, the main aim is to control, or suppress, the appetite. This is done firstly by reducing stomach acid production. Those who eat very fast, use a lot of chillies, drink a lot of orange, lemon ,pineapple ,white wine hot sauces, alcohol etc. have excess stomach acid. This increases the appetite. Secondly, by allowing the taste buds to function better, the feeling of satiety comes sooner and this suppresses the appetite. Thirdly, the neck massage helps to keep the glucose supply to the appetite centre under optimum control. Finally, my herbal teas suppress the appetite.

If the sugar level in the blood drops drastically, as in Hypoglycaemia, there is intense panic. The muscles shake violently to release stored glucose; cold sweats appear along with disorientation or fainting. One feels better if one lies down on the floor horizontally without a pillow. A lump of sugar cures it instantly. If that is not available, a neck and shoulder massage reduces the symptoms. The Hypothalamus stops sending panic signals and the body calms down. Lack of sugar in the brain causes intense emotional problems. You feel fear, anger, grief, panic etc in varying degrees of intensity.

Diabetics often get hypoglycaemic attacks. Even before it's diagnosed, people get cold sweats, fear, panic, tremors etc. They often do not understand why they get these symptoms. Once blood tests have been done, the diagnosis can be established. Those who inject insulin are more likely to get hypoglycaemia as the dosage may be difficult to judge sometimes.

* * * * *

A friend's secretary was desperate to lose weight. She lost her boyfriend, could not fit into her clothes and hated herself in the mirror. She had tried the Atkin's Diet; lost quite a bit, but put it back on when she stopped the programme. She couldn't keep up with her exercises as she became fatigued easily. Her boss and my friend asked her to see me.

She felt embarrassed, as she had to disclose her problems to me. She couldn't handle it.

Finally, one day she made an appointment to come and see me. She started talking about her ankle sprain and her backache. She said she got tired very easily and had occasional headaches. I went straight to the point: did she binge? She finally admitted that she craved sugar and sweets all the time and she had to have something sweet every hour. I tried to discover if she had any trauma to her head or neck. She couldn't recall anything, but admitted that she worked long hours in front of a computer and needed two pillows to sleep. These were the reasons for her fatigue and sugar cravings.

With an excuse to treat her neck and back, I gave her some treatment. After a couple of sessions, I asked her if her sugar cravings had reduced. Her eyes twinkled with surprise; the cravings had disappeared.

I explained why she had them and put her on my weight loss plan. Without her cravings, her weight dropped. She ate sensibly and was strong enough to go to the gym 2-3 times a week. She was ecstatic. Everyone, including me when she came to visit, started telling her how wonderful she looked. This boosted her morale enormously. She continued going to the gym regularly. The more weight she lost, the better she felt. It was difficult to believe that this lady had transformed herself so well. The sugar and food cravings had imprisoned her.

6.12 The Roles of Oxygen and Glucose

If lack of oxygen in the environment causes fatigue, headaches, dizziness, fainting etc over a few seconds, then lack of glucose in the blood, or hypoglycaemia, causes panic, emotional problems, shivering for a few minutes. The body has a reserve of glucose and so it tries desperately to release that. A sudden release of stored glucose eases the situation and acts as damage-control mechanism. It is when that reserve is exhausted that the body experiences serious symptoms.

Oxygen is mainly supplied to the brain by the blood, whereas glucose is also provided by the cerebro-spinal fluid (CSF) which bathes the brain. The CSF also circulates and so there is scope for more glucose to be available to the brain to fuel its activity.

During clinical fasting, patients undergo treatment for 15-20 days, or more, with just water and a little honey. No food is given to them and the body is forced to release fuel from stored fat in the body. Thus, lack of glucose in the brain tissue is not fatal but lack of oxygen has serious consequences. In an acute stroke, the body becomes paralysed on one side with loss of speech or swallowing, due to a clot in one or the other artery of the brain. This clot totally starves the corresponding area of oxygen, causing nerve cells to fail. This results in paralysis. Oxygen is absolutely essential for the functioning of the brain cells.

6.13 Bell's Palsy

This is a condition where one half of the face becomes paralyzed. The eye is wide open, the angle of the mouth drops on one side, there is constant drooling on the affected side as the mouth cannot shut and the tongue is forked to one side.

This happens as a result of the loss of function in the facial nerve or 7th Cranial nerve, which originates in the midbrain. Most physicians, or neurologists, think that the condition is a viral infection of the facial nerve. Sometimes it is considered to be due to inflammation of the nerve due to a cold draft on that side of the face.

This nerve is fairly thick, originating in the midbrain, and emerging out of the cranium or skull, through a small hole located in front of the ear. The nerve then divides into several branches. This is the main nerve for the facial, or mimicry muscles, controlling one's expression. A part of the nerve picks up information from the taste buds in the anterior part of the tongue (which tastes both sweet and salty flavours). Besides this, the branches of the facial nerve control the secretion of tears, mucus discharge in the nose and salivary secretion.

My hypothesis is that the Basilar Artery, which is formed by the joining of the two vertebral arteries on the left and right sides, gives out branches to feed the roots of the facial nerves. These blood vessels are tiny and are called vasa nervorum (vessels of the nerve). All nerves are fed by these tiny blood vessels.

When the pressure of the blood in the Basilar Artery drops, due to constriction in the vertebral arteries, the vasa nervorum receives very little blood. This impairs the function of the facial nerve and the result is Bell's Palsy.

It is very frightening, as within a few minutes, half of the face becomes non-functional. It is not a stroke, as no clot in the corresponding arteries can be seen. It is just that one major nerve has lost its function. No one has ever found a virus in the nerve, but I have all the proof necessary to confirm that it is due to impaired blood flow to the facial nerve. By restoring the blood flow with massage of the facial muscles, along with exercises, the functions have been restored in hundreds of cases.

* * * * *

Tom Chapman, the son of my close family friends Frank and Wendy Chapman woke-up one morning with his face paralysed on one side. The worst symptom was his inability to close his eyelid on the affected side . He went to his doctor who prescribed him steroids, as the nerve was inflamed. He said he would do anything, for three months to three years, to resolve the problem. He panicked because he was in the fashion business and had to deal with elite customers. Tom owned 'Matches' a well known luxury chain for clothes in London.

Tom came to see me late that night at home. I reassured him that he would be alright and explained what had happened. It was true that he had been extremely stressed and because of the business, he had an unhealthy lifestyle, travelled a lot and slept badly. His neck was very stiff, which I treated along with his facial muscles and I gave him some exercises. I saw him regularly for a few weeks and the symptoms disappeared. I saw the first improvement in the eye, which is something patients are always most concerned about. At first you can sleep with your eye open. Then, if the eyelids don't move, the 'wipers' of the eye are non-functional. All sorts of dust from the atmosphere settles on it and the chances of an eye infection are very high. You have to wear an eye patch to prevent this from happening.

* * * * *

A film director from Darjeeling was in Delhi. I was there on holiday. Someone brought him over to see me. He was a wonderful man but Bell's Palsy had destroyed his life. He was very depressed, as six months had passed without any improvement. He was very concerned that producers didn't give him any work.

In those days, some twenty-eight years ago, I had not discovered the 'Neck Connection'. I began to give him acupuncture and to massage his face, along with the area behind the ears and some pressure points on the neck. I did not have enough experience, as I may have only come across one or two patients in Moscow, where I had completed my post graduation in Acupuncture.

The treatment worked with this patient. He took several weeks to recover and he was eventually cured. Today, when I look back at this case, I can clearly see how acupuncture helped. It not only improved the blood flow to the nerve, but also stimulated it. The treatment must have generally boosted his energy and he was able to heal without much effort.

Prior to each treatment he drank pigeon soup and massaged his face with a little clove oil, which has a heating effect on the muscles and nerves. Clove is 'hot' oil, and is the traditional treatment for paralysis. The pigeon soup also 'heated' the body and the nerves. Paralysis is considered to be a 'cold' disease and the cure is to 'heat' the body.

* * * * *

The President of a major world institution was travelling a lot and was very exhausted. One afternoon he told his secretary to cancel his post-luncheon appointments as he was very tired and didn't have the energy to meet anyone. He lay on the sofa in his large office and slept with a cushion under his neck. Within minutes he drifted-off into a deep sleep.

When he woke-up, one half of his face felt strange. He got-up and felt dizzy and imbalanced. He called his secretary who was shocked to see him. He was pale in the face, his facial expression on one side had gone and the facial muscle had drooped. She immediately called the emergency services.

The helicopter ambulance landed on the top of his office block and he was taken to the best hospital in Washington DC. A CT scan and all investigation were done. There was nothing significantly wrong with his brain and heart. It was a classic case of Bell's Palsy.
Steroids were prescribed and physiotherapy was recommended. With rest, his fatigue improved, but the face remained lop-sided. The word spread and the Chinese Government sent their best acupuncturist, as he was very important for the development of their country in the nineties and he was a very well-respected leader of the world institution.

The acupuncturist treated him for five weeks, following him around on his plane. His face improved slightly and he was able to partially close his eyes. He didn't feel right about his condition, as he was a public figure and was photographed frequently. Most people who met him asked him how he was doing and he found that embarrassing.

A senior member of the British Royal Family met him in his Washington office for some work. Seeing him, he immediately recommended me. He very kindly sang my praises and described my work with stroke research at The Hammersmith Hospital in London, using my technique. I received a call to say that I would be called from the office of this important gentleman in Washington who had Bell's Palsy.

I was in Geneva, in the beautiful Beau Rivage Hotel, when I received the call from Washington. The gentleman explained what had happened and asked if I treated a late case of Bell's Palsy, as five months had already passed and he had not fully recovered. His eye still did not shut properly and it watered. I told him about my theory and technique and he found my explanation quite satisfactory. He wanted to fly me over to Washington DC. I explained that I was treating someone in

Geneva and would be available next week. He said he would try to fly over to London to see me over the weekend.

On the following Friday evening, I received a call to say that his plane could not take-off due to heavy snow fall. He suggested that I flew to New York the following weekend and go on to join him in Aspen, Colorado, where he would be available for four days. He had no major appointments, other than to sit on a panel, and would be available for five days in all for treatment. This was the only clear slot in his diary.

I flew to New York, had supper with him in his beautiful apartment and went to La Guardia airport. On his plane, after take-off, I began to treat him on his bed, as I did not want to waste any time. Being a small Lear jet, it was slightly cramped, but I had adequate space to treat his neck, face and then his entire body for two hours or so.

His neck muscles were extremely tight, as I expected. He too was very surprised as no one had ever noticed this. I could feel that a couple of vertebrae in his neck were misaligned. I worked deeply and warned him that he would bruise slightly because of the treatment. Time was short and I had to condense the treatments. When I treated his back and his legs, he felt relaxed and fell asleep. I was then able to recline in my seat and relax.

We stayed in the house of Evelyn and Leonard Lauder, the cosmetic giant. They were such a wonderful couple. The following morning, my patient came down and said he felt slightly better in the face and certainly more energetic. The improved blood flow to the brain had done the trick.

We went to the conference venue. Ted Forstman, whose family owned the Gulf Stream, organised this conference every year and invited all the owners for a three day event. Major speakers were invited to share their views on the economy, politics, environmental issues etc. I met many world statesmen and important people there. The conference was fabulously organised and the speakers were excellent. I learnt so much from the discussions. Then there was a surprise! President Nelson Mandela was linked via satellite and he spoke to us from Cape Town. That made my day, as I adore Mandela.

After lunch, I would go for walks with Leonard and Evelyn in the wild mountains.

With renewed energy and a refreshed mind, I treated my lovely patient twice a day. Whilst he was bruised, his confidence grew. He saw the truth behind the 'Neck Connection'. He had seen the best doctors and had received the best treatment. My approach, although not scientifically proven, had a logical explanation.

I managed to treat him again on the plane. I showed him all the exercises; drew the diagrams for his physiotherapists, so that he could continue his treatment. He did come over to London a couple of times and I gave him treatment in his hotel. His condition steadily improved. In his case, the physiotherapy and acupuncture made the initial improvement but that soon reached a plateau and he made no further progress. My technique and treatment pushed the progress up from the plateau. I wish I had seen him right from the beginning, and then he would not have had to go through that agony for so many months.
From time to time, I have seen his photograph in magazines and I study his facial expressions. It did look almost alright, except for a slight droop in the angle of his mouth.

6.14 Ageing

T. S. Eliot, the famous poet, wrote: *My life is light, waiting for the death wind, like a feather on the back of my hand.* This concept of playing out time has become out dated as technology has put power into the hands of the Elderly. As a result the population of the elderly is growing in the West. There is no "medicine" for the elderly, preventative or therapeutic. All we have is Geriatric Medicine, available to people who are overcome with illnesses of the aged.
Having dealt with very many elderly people, I feel many of their problems are largely preventable. In a nutshell, they need to eat differently, as their digestive enzymes are no longer available in abundance, and their stomach and intestinal muscles lose the ability to churn or contract as before. Softer foods and a very light dinner eaten at sunset, or shortly afterwards is highly recommended.

My neck treatment helps to keep all the vital centres functional at an optimal level. They are able to sustain the energy level, maintain balance and coordination of gait, digest better, prevent dizziness, severe insomnia, neck stiffness, tinnitus, blurred vision, tremor in the hands and vision deterioration.

* * * * *

A lady in her 80s had Macular Degeneration with reduced central vision. She had fatigue, dizziness and imbalance. The neck treatment improved Blood Flow to the Optic Nerve and improved her vision such that she could see faint figures on the TV. She can now walk without feeling dizziness and her energy is a lot better. She visits the clinic from time to time to maintain her vision and balance.

* * * * *

William Kessler, a man in his 80s, has been seeing me at the clinic at regular intervals. His dizziness, imbalance, short term memory, tinnitus and fatigue are kept under control with the neck treatments , and whenever there is a gap in the treatments the symptoms come back, and he makes an appointment immediately. We have become great friends over the years. He has been on my Himalayan trips, several times, and has greatly benefited from the treatments at the altitude. He often tells me that my discovery of the Vertebral Arteries' role in well-being and self-healing deserves a big research and recognition for its contribution to medicine. He says that it is the safest, cheapest and the most beneficial single treatment in the world. It has a cure-all effect on the body as healing is a deeper function of Nature. Once aroused in the body, everything else follows automatically.

* * * * *

Bill Bruce, a friend of mine, whom I had not seen for a while, came to see me at the clinic. I immediately noticed his slurred speech. He was surprised that I noticed it and his doctors didn't even do so, though he complained about it. He said he had come to see me for his imbalance and dizziness. I checked him up, and he had many symptoms of the Ali Syndrome as well as an extremely stiff and immobile neck.

I began to see him once a week. He would fly down from Aberdeen, and stay overnight at the club so that he could have two sessions per week. Gradually, his gait and his imbalance improved. I took him to the Spa in Tuscany, and he followed a strict programme of diet, neck massage, walking and yoga. His condition has improved noticeably. Given his age, I have asked him to see me from time to time to control his condition. He looks much younger, the energy level is good, he sleeps well, his memory has improved, his digestion and bowel evacuation has improved and he no longer has any joint stiffness. It has changed his life. From feeling old and "Rusty" as he called it. He is very energetic now, and works very hard.

There are other additional benefits from having regular neck treatments in old age. People generally feel very energetic, and so they can walk and carry out their routine work. They suffer from less colds and coughs as the immune system improves. I have noticed changes on the skin as well. With treatment, the ageing process slows down. The most significant change is the increased level of energy and improved memory, something that elderly people long to maintain in their system.

Women who suffer from osteoporosis, usually lose calcium from the neck region and the hips or pelvic bones. As a result of that they lose height. The discs in the neck degenerate and facilitate the "shrinkage". This causes the vertebral canals to deform as well, resulting in poor blood flow in the vertebral arteries. They feel extremely tired and complain of constant neck tension. That is followed by headaches and dizziness or vertigo, nausea, imbalance etc.

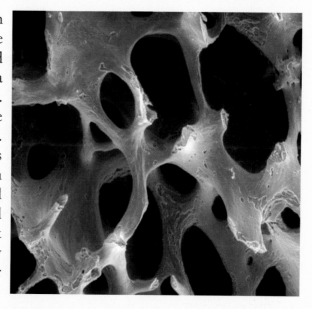

* * * * *

The widow of a leading Russian musician, known very well in the West, was wheelchair-bound. She had no power in her legs and couldn't walk due to severe imbalance. She herself was a very famous singer and ran a school in central Moscow. I was introduced to her by a well-known Russian musician living in the West. I went back to Moscow after 25 years and was very emotional. A lot had changed, and it was a new country, quite different from what it was when I left in 1982 after my post graduation.

On the first day I went to the Moscow Conservatory, where this amazing lady received the Tchaikovsky award, given posthumously to her late husband. She walked with a couple of men supporting her to receive the award on the stage. The imbalance was severe.

I worked on her neck and back. After three days of treatment, she got her strength back. She was able to walk unaided, and no longer used the wheelchair. After a few days, I went back to see her and completed a course of treatment. She was back at work at her singing school.

* * * * *

A friend's mother lived in Henley, near London. She could not walk as she had extreme fatigue, dizziness, imbalance and arthritis. She had a fall and broke her neck. Although the bones healed, she continued to have many of the symptoms of the Ali Syndrome. A specialist had warned her that she must not let anybody touch her neck. I told my friend to bring her to me.

I asked a colleague who treats patients at home to visit her twice a week. I told her to focus on the neck and shoulder. After just a month's treatment the elderly lady came to see me at the clinic. She was walking without support. Her energy too had improved. The quality of her life improved dramatically. Because of her age, she was told she would have to live with it. But now she is enjoying her life.

Some arteries form plaque on the inner surface due to cholesterol deposit. In old age it can become worse. It is not the misaligned vertebrae, which cause the problem, but the narrowing of the artery, which reduces the blood flow. In such cases the tinnitus, imbalance and TIA (mini-stroke like symptoms) are often common phenomena. A strict fat-free diet, neck massage, exercises and sleeping on a very flat pillow help the situation. The replacement of this damage is a very risky surgery. Any complication will have fatal consequences.

It is my dream to operate A Fractional Ownership Complex for the Elderly, where people between the age of 60 and 90 years could buy a unit for 1 to 3 months a year. These units would be self sufficient. They would have easily accessible facilities, like common dining room, swimming pool, therapies section, recreational section, multi-faith prayer hall, etc. Each resident would receive 2 to 3 sessions of neck and body massage per week, attend aerobatic and elderly yoga exercises and eat as per individual requirement in the dining hall. Thus each person owning the unit would have 1 to 3 months of health care with diet, massage, exercises and walks in the fresh air. They could resolve their aches and pains, improve their digestive system, relax and sleep well. Moreover, activities like film clubs, lectures, dancing classes, excursions, painting, etc, would also stimulate their brains.

They could own units for up to 30 years, but would pay a yearly service charge for maintenance as well, as for their meals, treatments and extras. There would be a doctor on duty for 24 hours to attend to any emergency calls.

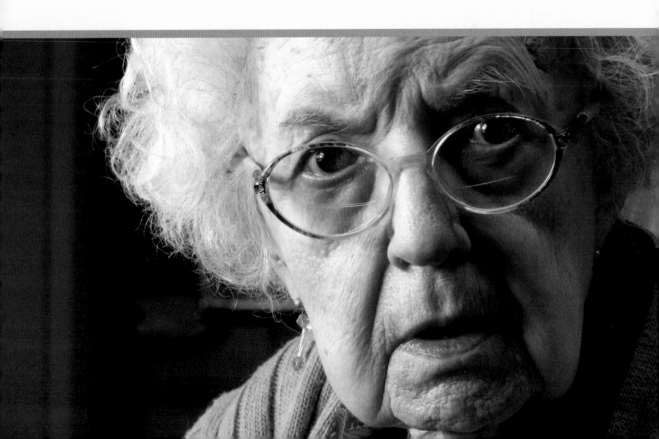

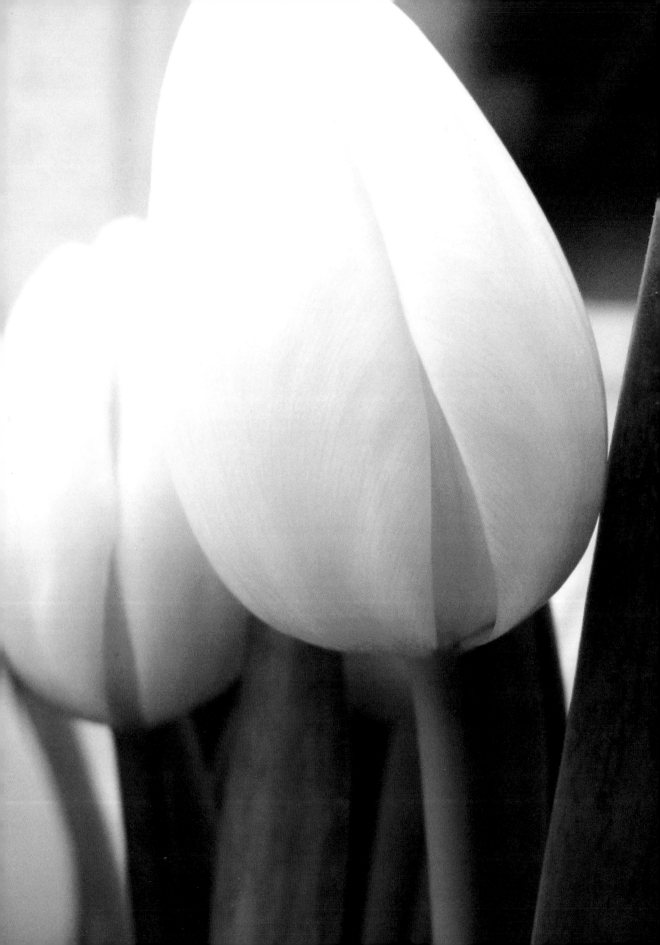

PART 2

Case Histories

T I A (Transient Ischaemic Attack)

This is often regarded as a 'mini stroke' or a 'transitory stroke'. It has all the symptoms of a stroke, like weakness in one half- side of the body with Facial paralysis on the opposite side (if the arm and leg are paralyzed on the left, the face will be paralyzed on the right), loss of speech (if right side of body is paralyzed), extreme fatigue etc. The only difference is that it does not last long. Within a few hours or days the recovery takes place, sometimes without any treatment.

For the patient or the family, it is very scary . Sometimes the attacks occur every so often and the patient is extremely anxious. As scans show no noticeable change in the brain it is often not considered to be serious by doctors. There may not be a second attack and there is spontaneous recovery. It is considered to be a spasm of the arteries and there is no clot formation. The spasm causes a decreased blood flow to the brain.

A TIA in the vertebral artery causes extreme fatigue, fainting, loss of vision, near death experience like falling into an abyss or tunnel and other psychological phenomena. The body may not suffer from any paralysis or weakness. It often sorts itself out when a patient is laid flat on the back. The horizontal position, helps blood to flow to the brain and the patient recovers. The TIA is often confused with Vaso-Vagal reaction as the lack of blood supply to the Vagus nerve center in the brainstem is considered to be the primary cause. Vagus nerve controls breathing and heart beat. When they stop, fainting occurs.

* * * * *

Once I was on my way to Muscat via Abu Dhabi. We were flying over Iran on a British Airways flight. I was sleeping on my bed in front when there was an announcement on the PA system. They were paging for a doctor immediately. I responded by pressing the call button. A stewardess took me to the Business class section. An Asian gentleman was slumped in his seat with the face distinctly dropped on one side . He was unconscious.

I laid him down on the aisle and stretched his neck. I found a few dis-aligned vertebrae in the neck and began to gently adjust them. Within a couple of minutes, he revived. He tried to get up as he was very embarrassed at what had happened. I told him to lie on his back. We cleared the area between the club world seats (in those days BA had cradle seats and not flat bed) and put him there, with just a blanket under his head and no pillows.

I asked his wife if he had neck problems. She confirmed that he always complained of dizziness and neck pain. I massaged his neck, opened his collar buttons and gave him some water to drink. After a few minutes he fell asleep. His wife said that he was very exhausted in the previous few days and he complained of headaches.

I went back to my seat and told the wife to let me know when he woke up. Shortly afterwards the captain called me to the cockpit. He asked me what was wrong with the passenger. I explained that his neck was stiff and it cut off blood supply to the brain, causing him to collapse. Additionally, the facial nerve reacted and so there was loss of facial expression on one side. I adjusted the vertebrae of the neck and reinstated the blood flow which revived him. He asked me if he needed to order an ambulance or medical team prior to our arrival. I said I would let him know, when we started our descent. I had suggested that landing in Tehran, as he was intending to do, would not have been a good idea.

The captain ordered tea for me gave me the duty free booklet. He asked me to choose as many items I wanted to take as a token of thanks. I was quite surprised. I chose a small teddy for the daughter of a relative. The captain asked me again and again to choose some perfumes or ties but I didn't feel I should, I just did my duty.

TIA is usually experienced in the carotid artery but if it happens on the vertebral arteries then fainting and fits are common symptoms. This is because the vital centers in the brain stem are deprived of blood. As that happens the breathing and heartbeat switch off momentarily and so one is unconscious.

* * * * *

The collapse of George Bush senior at a press conference in Tokyo I considered to be a TIA or Vaso-Vagal reaction. He was exhausted from the long flight from Washington DC to Tokyo, had a hectic schedule and probably suffered terrible jet lag. Thus in front of the camera in full view of world media and with live broadcast world wide, he collapsed and threw up. It was an embarrassing moment and everyone was alarmed. Once he was on the floor with the head positioned horizontally, the blood flow to the brain was reinstated and he regained consciousness. He was hospitalized and investigation showed that he had slightly high thyroid function. I cannot believe that hyperthyroidism, which generally causes panic and palpitation, would make him collapse unless the heart failed. In my opinion it was TIA, or Vaso-Vagal reaction.

* * * * *

A British Prime Minister, also fainted and collapsed during his tenure. He was over exhausted and probably had some palpitation as well. According to the Press release he had irregular heart beat for which a surgical procedure (ablation) was performed in the electrical conductive fibres inside the heart. He must have been on medication. In this case the irregular heart beat meant that his heart was not pumping enough blood to the brain. The reason he collapsed was that he probably had a very tight neck in addition and the blood flow to the vital centers of the midbrain was so poor that they stopped functioning momentarily (Transient Ischaemic Attack).

* * * * *

One of the most severe cases of this attack I experienced was that of a professor in Oxford University. He used to collapse frequently during lectures especially when he was tired. He would lose control of his muscles of the leg and spine and slump on the dais. He had seen many specialists and no one could pin point the problem. He came to see me in London. I really felt sorry for him as it must have been very embarrassing to collapse in front of his students.

The professor did suffer from a very tight neck and sometimes felt nervous before the lecture. He didn't have any control over the attack and was taken by surprise every time it happened. I explained the situation and demonstrated how the neck massage was done. I suggested that he saw someone regularly for a deep tissue massage in Oxford as the journey to London was almost an hour and was too strenuous for him. I showed him a set of yoga exercises.

I wanted to follow up this case as it was the first and only one that showed such dramatic reaction to lack of blood flow to the brain. In Private Medicine, however, it's sometimes very difficult as people are concerned about their finances. Even if you offer them free consultation, they are reluctant or embarrassed to be treated.

This professor had all the telltale signs of Ali Syndrome – fainting or collapsing, slight dizziness, long hours in front of the computer, fatigue, insomnia etc. He had all the tests and scans to rule out a brain tumour, viral encephalitis, atrophy of brain tissue etc. It was nothing but Transient Ischaemic Attack, or temporary attack of reduced blood supply to the brain caused by neck stiffness, aggravated stress and a stuffy auditorium with poor ventilation. He was told it was a psychological problem which he strongly denied. This was the conflict he faced in his mind.

CHAPTER 8

Hysteria

Though not strictly an example of the Ali Syndrome, the treatment for hysteria can be closely related. A few years ago I was training some NHS doctors in the Principles of Integrated Medical Diagnosis and Treatment. We were in the Himalayas. One day, a medical camp was set up in a remote primary healthcare center for the doctors to examine the patients independently. When we arrived some 300 patients showed up and we were 8 doctors in all. The rumours had spread in the hills that some doctors from England were holding a free medical camp so they walked miles from their villages for consultations. My students were shocked when they found they faced such a mammoth task.

We started consultations immediately. I saw a patient every 3 minutes as sending them back home without even a brief chat would have been disheartening for them. Many were jumping the queue as they were so anxious. Some had arrived early in the morning to get a ticket with a number so they could be part of a queue.

Suddenly, two of our doctors rushed to me saying there was an emergency, explaining a woman had collapsed in the crowd. I waded through the throng and reached her. She was put on the veranda as there was no bed. I looked at her and found her teeth clenched but she was breathing - only just. From experience I instantly knew what the case was. I turned to the doctors, who had by then gathered there to help. 'What do you think has happened?' I asked.

They said we should take her to the nearest hospital as the primary healthcare center was not equipped. They felt the pulse, it was there. She was breathing slowly. I was calm and wanted them to see this very interesting case - but they were panicking as they thought she would die right in front of them.

I asked them to come nearer and watch me treat her. I told everybody to be silent.

I asked for a spoon and with it I forcefully opened her clenched teeth. They saw it was really tight. I pressed the two points in the center of the forehead, on the top of the bridge of the nose. Usually, these trigger points, or pressure points, are very sensitive. When I pressed hard she blinked a little. I told them to observe that she responded to pain.

I moved close to her and in Hindi, told her softly that she would be cured. I almost whispered in her ears. I said I knew what her problems were and her body would become better again. I could see that the doctors were losing their patience. They had seen mini miracles during their training programme where I showed them with accurate diagnosis, instant treatments but my casual approach to a patient in 'coma' as irritating. I smiled at them and continued to talk to her. I stroked her head and massaged her jaw and the neck.
After 5 minutes of talking and using caring words, she opened her eyes. The doctors began to clap and were overjoyed. They were awed by the whole incident. How could I talk her out of coma? I gave the patient some water to drink and she sat up.

I called the doctors to one side and asked the medical officer of the health center to join me. I explained what had happened, namely that it was a typical case of hysteria. We all know what being 'hysterical' means but that was a hysterical attack.

* * * * *

In ancient times, Greek Medicine, led by Hippocrates and later by Galen, this condition was called 'hysteria' or twisting of the uterus (hystericus-uterus; hysterectomy-removal of uterus). Women who have unfulfilled sexual desire, or who do not get an orgasm after severe arousal, can experience disappointment and frustration. They may bottle up their feelings to avoid conflict with their husband or partner. If this happens repeatedly they develop this psychological condition. It is a great 'drama' as it tends to happen in the presence of a crowd or in family gatherings. Hysterical attacks never happen when these women are on their own. In honeymoon periods in conservative countries like India, Middle East, China etc, when young girls first experience sexual encounters, they often don't know what an orgasm is. They are nervous and confused by the speeding heart rate, excessive sweating, tensed muscles, panic breathing etc. Very often they get tremors and shakes. Initially, doctors are called in but most feel embarrassed as it is linked to sex. This tension grows and they get these uncomfortable attacks where they faint and become very tensed. They can hear everything around but cannot move. They respond to pain and smooth talking only. Giving them oxygen or putting a drip in is not going to help as it is purely psychological but causes great anxiety to the people observing them.

The doctors were so surprised that they started laughing. Moments before that they had been in great fear and their call-of duty demanded that they do something immediately. Resuscitation was not needed as she was breathing and had pulse.

* * * * *

In the modern world women are sexually liberated and have gradual personal experience. Sex education takes away the myth and they know everything about it. In underdeveloped societies, such facilities are not available. Sex is a taboo subject. Young girls learn from married friends, elder sisters or grandmothers. Some don't have that opportunity and they are more likely to get hysteria.

When people faint suddenly one has to take into account some common factors. The cause could be due to anemia or very low blood pressure, hypoglycemia or low blood sugar, extreme fatigue and dehydration, high blood sugar (for a known diabetic), epileptic fits (when the person has a seizure), stroke etc. The vast majority do so because of a neck condition. So if you see someone collapse in a crowded place, make the person lie on their back. Clear the area of crowd so that there is fresh air. Massage the neck and give it a gentle traction. Give them some water to drink when they turn around and are conscious. Keep them lying on their backs while you call for medical help for a definite diagnosis. Most people will recover and walk home.

Stroke

This is another extreme condition of total lack of blood flow in one of the arteries of the brain. It is caused by a clot in the blood that travels from the heart and is pushed up towards the brain. In a majority of cases the clot travels along the wider Carotid artery and continues to travel along the length of it till it gets stuck in the narrower blood vessel of the conscious brain and plugs it, causing total loss of blood flow to the corresponding area of the cortical or conscious brain. Depending on where the clot is and how much area of the brain it cuts out, the damage can be substantial. Typically, a small clot in that arterial network will cause loss of power in opposite side of the body, paralysis of the same side of the face (because the nerves from the brain cross over from one side to the other side at the level of the upper neck), loss of sensation etc.

If a clot is large in size then a large part of the brain gets shut off. The result is a devastating stroke. The patient is unconscious and one half of the body is totally paralyzed with less hope of recovery using conventional methods. If the clot affects the right side of the brain, there is loss of speech. Speech and writing are connected. If the person is a right-hander, a left-sided stroke will destroy speech. Remember nerves from the right side of the brain cross over to the left side of the body and vice versa.

The conscious or cortical brain is responsible for sensation, voluntary movement, vision, speech analysis, logic, decision making etc. Much of it gets affected, depending on how large a clot it is. Fortunately, the other half of the brain is spared in a single stroke and so higher functions like long-term memory, recognition, analysis of the situation, communication with eyes or partial expression (if speech is gone) etc are intact or partially intact.

A stroke often shuts off the brain suddenly and so one looses consciousness, depending on the size of the clot and where the blood circulation has stopped. There is often a swelling in the brain which affects the circulation of brain fluids. This in turn causes loss of consciousness, difficulty in breathing, swallowing etc. A drip is put in to re-hydrate the brain with steroids and other medicines as swallowing, a voluntary act is affected. Thus a feeding tube is inserted. It is because of the increase in brain fluid pressure, a part of the skull is removed in the hope that the pressure will not damage the brain surface substantially.

If the clot is small and misses the Carotid Artery in front of the neck, it might be pushed into the vertebral artery. This has a devastating effect, especially if the clot is large enough to block the basilar (formed by the union of the vertebral arteries, (see diagram) artery.

This means the vital centres' of the brain are shut out. This leads to instant death. A smaller clot can sneak through to cause lesser damage like loss of vision (optic nerve damage on one side) in one eye, lack of balance, vertigo, etc. Most strokes in the vertebral arterial network are fatal. This once again proves my point. Without the vertebral arteries our existence is not possible.

Why am I talking about stroke when it is caused by a clot and not due to constriction of the artery due to a neck problem? It has relevance here because my Stroke Rehabilitation Technique uses the vertebral arteries to supply vital brain fluid to the areas that can be reached. Thus the brain tissue, which is not affected by the stroke, can be kept going with supply of glucose and some oxygen. The vertebral arterial network may also open up some collateral to the areas close to the stroke-affected area (via Internal Carotid artery- see fig. 3). These areas take up the functions of the destroyed or dead areas of the brain that had its blood supply cut off. Vertebral arteries help the formation of cerebrospinal fluid which bathes the brain. The exudates from some branches of the Vertebro-basilar arteries form CSF.

Improving blood supply to the subconscious part of the brain restores such functions as breathing, heart rate, digestion, appetite, general well being, improved energy, emotions, sleep, swallowing etc. This goes a long way in the general rehabilitation. It gives you the strength to go through the physical therapies and improves your participation in it. After a major shock to the system, the subconscious brain creates a certain amount of alertness and positive emotions to face the situation and recover. The 'will to fight' is a major stimulus.

(OLFACTORY BULB FOR SMELL)

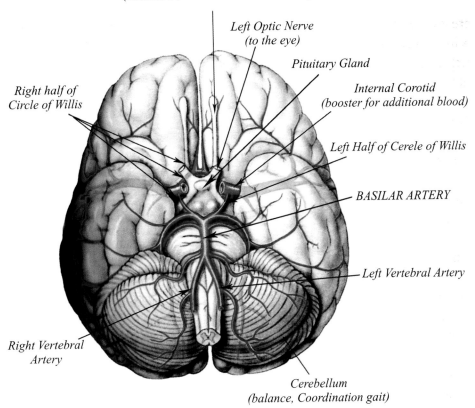

Fig. 3

Blood Vessels (Arteries) on the inferior Surface of the brain

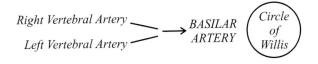

Having treated hundreds of stroke victims and helped them to lead a near normal life has given me some authority to speak about Stroke Rehabilitation using The Ali Technique.

* * * * *

Angie Gooderham, a friend in her fifties went with me to India over the Christmas-New Year period. My mother joined me on that trip. We traveled by train to Ajmer, where we visited our family's Sufi saint's shrine, offered prayers and drove to my friend's Bijaipur castle in a remote part of eastern Rajasthan. That used to be my winter retreat until it became a very popular heritage hotel. I used to walk through the jungles looking for herbs, watching hundreds of species of birds, visiting tribal settlements to see their lives from close quarters and going on game drives with search light at night. I learnt so much about nature from being there. I learnt about lives of ancient tribes.

After arrival we went to the terrace to look at the moon, which had a strange but large halo around it. I saw Angie in tears and asked her if she was alright. She didn't reply so I thought she was overwhelmed by the peace and beauty of that 300 year old castle. I went down to the courtyard of the castle to have tea with my friend Rao Narender Singh, the owner of the castle.

One of my therapists came down quickly to tell me that a lady was poorly and was lying in her bed. I rushed up to her suite and upon one look I could tell that she had had a stroke that affected the right side of the body. I made the instantaneous decision to treat her immediately. The nearest hospital was in Chittorgarh, about 40 kms and Udaipur, the nearest big city was 135 kms away. Transporting her in that condition would have had its own difficulty and we would have lost her.

I began to work on the neck while my assistant worked on the Marma points, that I had discovered helped to stimulate brain centers. Within a few minutes I could see the change in colour of her face. She looked better. I went downstairs to try to arrange a drip, as she looked very dehydrated. I asked my assistant to continue the treatment.

After two hours of therapy, there was a jerk in her right leg. She could move her leg. She indicated that she wanted to go to the toilet. To my great joy and surprise, she got up to go to the toilet .It was about 10 pm. I couldn't arrange a drip as it was too late and we were in a remote village. Using a spoon we made her drink some water, she could swallow – that was a great relief.

My sister- in- law Uzma who is a doctor was also there. She offered to stay by her bedside and keep her under observation. I went down to see my mother and, being a very gentle and caring person, she was terribly worried. I tried to tell her that everything was under control.

Next morning, with some help Angie came down four flights steps to a room on the ground floor .It was Christmas day. She had lost her speech but could just about use her right hand with the therapy. It wasn't even 16 hours after a massive stroke and there she was sitting up in bed and smiling. She handed over a piece of paper in which she wrote a Christmas greeting for me. What she wrote didn't make sense but she thought she wrote 'Merry Christmas'. Some word like flavour (flower) morning (merry), Coming (Christmas) didn't make any sense. That was quite amazing.

Uzma, having worked in emergency wards, handled the case very well. She established a drip, gave her some blood thinners, plenty of fluids and organized my physical therapy every 6 hours. My mother made pigeon soup, a traditional remedy for stroke in India. She must have learnt from her doctor father. She also massaged her feet using some form of reflexology treatment.

The patient began to improve every day. On New Year's Eve, Rao, the owner of the castle, had organized a dance performance by the Kalbelia tribe and she got up to dance with him. I was in tears as it was one of the success stories of my life.

When she returned, her friend received her at the airport and took her straight to St. Mary's hospital in London. A CT scan was immediately done. There was a tennis ball size stroke and the brain was massively damaged. She had atrial fibrilllation (irregular and rapid heart beat) which churned up the clot in the heart and sent it straight up to the left side of the brain. I remembered that she was dehydrated. She did not drink water for the whole day as Indian public toilets in those days, including the first class train coach, weren't clean at all. The dehydration caused the irregular heart beat and the clot.

The doctor at St. Mary's could not believe that she was walking and speaking so soon after such a massive stroke. She called me to ask me how that happened. She wanted to know more about my treatment so I invited her to come to the clinic. She never came. Interestingly Angie lost her speech in French completely. She just forgot how to speak. It took years for that to come back.

* * * * *

About 8 years ago, I was training a batch of NHS doctors in Bijaipur Castle. One morning we went to the Chittorgarh General hospital for a tour to see the conditions in Indian hospitals. We were taken to the Intensive care unit, as it was pretty well equipped (basic according to UK standard). In one corner lay an old man who had had a stroke that morning and was admitted. A scan was performed earlier and the doctor in charge said he had no chance of survival. I asked him and the son of the patient if I could treat him using my hands only. They both agreed.

The patient was semi-conscious but was breathing independently. I worked on his neck and shoulders using my technique. The patient opened his eyes and had tears in his eyes. The son was ecstatic. My students, the doctors from UK, had their eyes glued on what was I doing.

Then I began to work on the Marma points in the right foot and leg. He jerked his left leg. I heard 'wow' behind me. I worked on his gluteal and back muscles, tested the power of his affected leg and made the patient sit up on the bed. I removed my hands and he was sitting without any support. The son was so happy. My students were very impressed with the 20 minutes treatment. The doctor in ICU, who was attending another serious patient in the ward, came running to see the patient wide alert and sitting independently on the side of the bed.

That is the power of the neck treatment, and in this case my stroke rehabilitation technique was watched by a group of doctors.

* * * * *

Later that day, we went to the Jetla Mata Temple some 5 km away from Chittorgarh in Rajasthan. This temple, it is believed, has a goddess that heals stroke, polio and paralyzed victims. I took the doctors to this temple. There were hundreds of patients lying there on their own or with their family members by their side. It is amazing that some people actually get better and return home. Some don't and spend months hoping they will. The temple committee provides food and water. Every 2 hours there is beating of the drums, ringing of bells and mass singing. The whole temple area becomes alive with an amazing array of sounds. Whoever can, tries to get up and offer prayers to the goddess in the sanctum sanctorum .The doctors found this fascinating.

I walked around with them and they observed the degree of disability some had. I spoke to several of them and narrated their personal story to my students. Amongst the many patients, I found a particular one who was on his own. An old man had had a stroke and he could only sit up. He was unmarried and lived on his own .His brother had left him several months ago, in the hope that either he would recover or become a permanent member there, waiting for his time. It was 'Aarti' time or prayer offering to the Gods.

I began to treat him and the doctors watched. They could see that with neck treatment, which had already convinced my doctors, as a powerful technique, and with massage of the affected limbs, the patient gained some power in them. After a while I held the hands of this patient and with some help from my students, I asked him to stand. To the surprise of many, he stood up. After a few minutes, I let go of his hands and he was able to stand independently. We helped him to walk a bit. There was commotion amongst the onlookers, as they wanted their relatives to be treated as well. It was getting late and we had to go back to the castle.

The following day, the doctors were very keen to go back and see what happened to the man. We drove to the temple and there he was sitting down and massaging his neck and the leg with the good hand. It was prayer time and as the music and songs started some people got up to dance and chant. To our surprise, our patient got up with great enthusiasm and began to dance.

A local TV crew had heard of the miracle of Chittorgarh General Hospital and, on reaching the temple, learnt that I was visiting there with a group of British doctors. They filmed the man dancing. It was a channel called E-TV (entertainment TV). They asked me to explain how this "miracle" happened. I spoke to them briefly. I wish I could have treated other patients but there were so many and selecting a few would have created a commotion amongst the others. I decided to leave with a sad heart feeling miserable that I could not reach out to them. I have since taken another group of doctors and the story was the same.

* * * * *

I used my stroke rehabilitation technique in three research projects. The first was at the Geriatric ward of the Hammersmith Hospital in Acton in 1996 under supervision of the then consultant, Dr. Mario Impalomeni, where 12 severely disabled patients with average age of 80.3 years were treated over a period of 5 months. The results amazed the team. Four walked with some aid and one walked independently. Another project was done under the supervision of The Peninsula Medical School in Exeter and carried out by my brother Nizam.. That study was published in The Journal of Physical Rehabilitation in 2006.

The third was done at Mayo Hospital, in Lucknow, India under supervision of consultant Dr. Sandip Aggarwal. Out of the selected 10 patients, 4 walked independently and 4 walked with a frame or stick. The Sahara group headed by our family friend Subroto Roy, sponsored the research and organized a press conference and the journalists were baffled by what they saw. Most newspapers carried the story the following day. Thousands of patients contacted the hospital after that. My nephew Ashique carried out the therapy.

I wish I had funding to carry out further research in this area. The research team in Exeter was very keen at one time to do a large nationwide study, but funding for rehabilitation is the least of the concerns of the Government. Unfortunately 40% of stroke victims are permanently disabled and 20% die. Only 40% regain some form of ability or are cured.

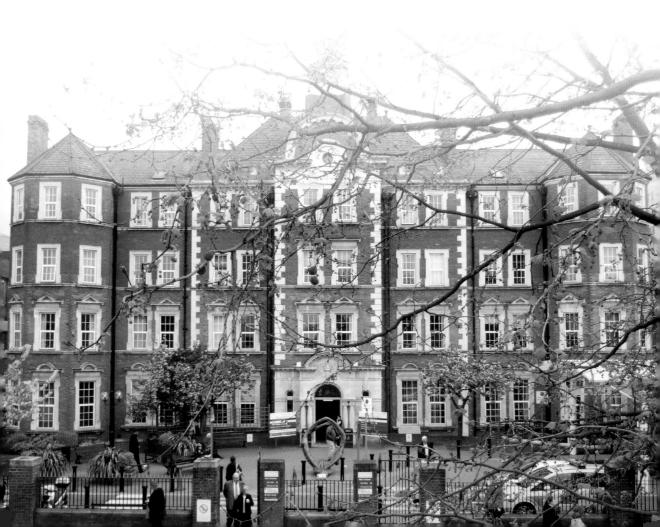

Coma

I worked in Delhi between 1982 and 1988 and established a good practice. Initially people were sceptical about my training and medical education in Moscow. They didn't understand Integrated Medicine. Acupuncture, Iridology, Yoga as therapy etc were outside their knowledge My fame came after success.

With help from Mrs. Sita Murari, the wife of Mr. Bob Murari, the then Secretary of The President of India, Central television filmed a 2- part documentary called, 'Search for an Alternative Cure'. They filmed me explaining what my system of Medicine was and showed my work with disabled patients. Three patients who were in coma for over six months and were discharged home came under my treatment. The TV team filmed their results.

A young man, the son of a Diplomat, was crossing the road when a speeding bus knocked him down. He was in AIIMS , India's leading research and teaching hospital for six months and was treated under eminent Neuro-physician Dr. Banerjee. When his condition was status quo, he was discharged home to spend rest of his life in that comatose state. His sister, a journalist heard of me and requested me to treat him. My assistant treated him using my technique. After only 8 weeks, the sister came to my clinic with a cassette recorder. She asked me to listen to the recording. It was my patient uttering his first words, quite incoherently .She was ecstatic. This patient went on to walk, talk and be quite independent. The lack of blood flow to the brain was the main problem because of neck trauma. The treatment simply reversed the process and the brain was rejuvenated again.

* * * * *

The daughter of a senior staff member in St. Columbus School (I studied in a similar Christian Brother's School, where I sometimes helped Mother Teresa in school holidays) went into a coma after a brain surgery to remove a tumor. She was fed through a tube but could breathe independently. She was sent home as nothing more could be done in the hospital. She remained in coma for 6 months until I was contacted. After 3 weeks of the treatment, she regained her consciousness. Then physical rehabilitation was carried out to make her walk. The TV interview showed her in perfectly normal condition.

* * * * *

A nun from the Brahma Kumari Organization, a well-known spiritual order, was involved in a head-on collision in Nepal. She was brought to Delhi and hospitalized. After 3 months, she was discharged, as her consciousness did not return. She was sent to their center in west Delhi. I examined her and decided to treat her. An assistant was designated to treat her daily. Some 4 weeks later, she regained consciousness but was still severely disabled due to various neurological injuries. Her first words were 'Om Shanti' the popular words used by Brahma-Kumaris to greet each other.

* * * * *

All these cases were demonstrated in a 2 part TV documentary broadcast on two consecutive days after the main English news bulletin at 9 pm. It was prime time and India's only channel then broadcasting to millions of homes. Within a couple of days thousands of patients, some in wheelchairs came to see me at The Center of Integrated Medicine in Delhi. I was stunned by the response the TV programme had. My landlord and the Housing Association, run by ex Army personnel got very alarmed. The lift was blocked, the residents complained and I was in serious trouble. The phone rang constantly. Finally, the Housing Association forcefully closed my clinic after an emergency meeting.

I desperately looked for alternative premises but no one was ready to let to me for fear that they would have to fight legal battles to evict me if I didn't voluntarily leave. After 2 months for search and with no place to practice from, I left India to take up a job at The Vital Life Centre in Hong Kong where I was already well-known, thanks to Aileen Bridgewater, a prominent radio talk show hostess who in just one interview on her Talk show made me famous overnight.

* * * * *

Another very interesting case of note was in Muscat, The Sultanate of Oman. The spiritual leader of a prominent tribe was driving home. He ate a piece of dry bread and choked. He collapsed in the car. His driver had the presence of mind to take him straight to the Royal Hospital, which was only a few minutes away. The excellent medical team resuscitated him and got his heart beating again. He was on ventilator, as he could not breathe independently.

Two months passed but there were no further signs of consciousness. His pupils were dilated and the doctors had no hope of reviving him, especially as he was 90 years old.

I was called in from London by His Majesty Sultan Qaboos bin Said Al Said as a last hope. Hundreds of Omani people dressed in astonishingly white robes stood outside the Royal Hospital and hoped for the best for their leader. It was quite an amazing sight.

I was taken to the Intensive Care Unit where I examined him. The team of doctors explained there was nothing that they could do and given his age and state, there was no hope for him. I explained my technique and said perhaps the improved blood flow through the vertebral arteries to the brain stem, where the vital centers of respiration and heart beat are, might just kick start the process of independent breathing. They had no clue as to what I was talking about because there was no reason for the blood to be obstructed in the vertebro-basilar arterial network. I explained that perhaps he hurt his neck when he collapsed in the car, as there was very little space available for him to fall. They were very nervous but took a written agreement from relatives and allowed me to treat him. I treated his neck in the ICU. A couple of days later one of my brothers, Firdous trained in the technique was flown in from Delhi to continue the treatment.

A month later he regained consciousness but spoke very little .The entire tribe rejoiced and the medical team was very surprised. He became very quiet in his 'second life' but he was conscious and ate normally.

I went to see a lady in Bangkok who was in a coma for eight years. She was breathing normally but was fed through the nasal Ryle's tube . She collapsed when she learnt that her husband had an affair with their Thai maid. They were Indian cloth merchants and rich.

I sent an assistant to treat her twice a day in the hospital. About 10 weeks later she regained full consciousness. My assistant had to go backward and forward for visa purpose. She became extremely quiet and had difficulty in walking. Six months later I went back to see her to give advise on physical rehabilitation. I was shocked to see her – she was all grey and had aged very quickly. For eight years, she froze in time and even looked younger. The worries of the world after gaining consciousness accelerated her ageing . That is why I advise meditation as a form of anti- ageing therapy.

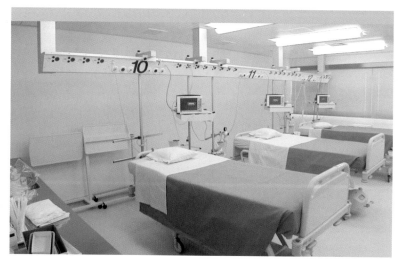

Complications of Birth Injuries

Birth injuries are becoming more common due to a variety of factors. Women do not prepare themselves for labour, especially if they work until the last minute. Socially, maternity leave is considered to be 'a sign of difference' from men. Many working women do not have much time for exercises, diet, and relaxation in the last trimester. Most tend to take the maternity leave after the baby is born. Women who do physical work in moderation have easier births.

If the birth canal is not ready or properly relaxed and the labour contractions are weak, the head is stuck at the entrance of the neck of the uterus for a long time. With each contraction the fragile neck of the baby is put under tremendous pressure. This is what happens in prolonged (over 15 hours) of labour.

If the contractions are vigorous, the baby's head opens up the tightened canal with great pressure and comes out in brief but rapid labour. This is what I call the 'champagne cork' birth. The head simply 'pops' out after less than 2 hours of labour.

In this case too, injuries to the neck are likely. The newborn baby has a very fragile neck, so it can't even support the neck. Imagine the trauma it goes through with such abnormal labour.

Forceps and Ventouse delivery causes the worse trauma to the head and neck of a newborn can face .The experienced hands of a qualified midwife could deliver babies in crisis perfectly. With the advance of medicine, the art has been replaced by technology. Stimulation, Suction, Caesarean operations are becoming common.

The umbilical cord around the neck can strangulate the baby. The cord is coiled around the neck and the labour force pushes the baby out. As the cord is of limited length, it squeezes the neck to allow the baby's exit out of the birth canal. If the labour is long then the trauma is intense. The baby is born blue. Depending on the severity and length of time the blood supply to the delicate brain is cut off, the extent of damage appears later in the baby's physical, emotional and physiological state.

Handling the baby after birth is also very important. You have to be extremely careful with the heavy head and a floppy neck. You simply can't hold the baby with one hand and do something with the other. You open the neck area to chance trauma especially as all the muscles and vertebrae are not fully developed. You have to be very careful during feeding time and especially while handling the head and neck area.

So many babies are born premature nowadays. Handling them is a delicate issue. They often sustain minor misalignments in the neck vertebrae, which are poorly joined at that stage. They are lying flat in the incubator. They are moved, fed, changed, turned etc and these do affect the delicate neck and head area where the fontanel's or bone free areas of the skull, are still wide open. All these make the neck and head very vulnerable to injury.

I can list a few of such complications that I observed in my years of practice.

11.1   Cerebral Palsy

This is a severe form of brain damage caused by strangulation of the two pairs of arteries supplying blood to the brain. Prolonged deprivation of blood to the brain is the primary cause of this devastating disease. It is often undiagnosed until a few months later when the child does not move the limbs or develops spasticity.

If the blood flow is reduced, for example due to the cord around the neck for 5-10 minutes during labour, the damage is very severe. There is loss of co-ordination of movement, spasticity in the limbs and the neck, loss of speech, learning difficulties etc. Some children show signs of high intelligence even if they cannot walk or move their hands in co-ordination. Society often has a negative attitude towards them. They can't move but the brain becomes sharp.

Upon interview, I found that the vast majority of them had cord around their neck, were born premature, had forceps delivery or some trauma sustained at labour. Some may have some genetic predisposition but that does not convince me.

* * * * *

The son of a Delhi industrialist was born with a cord around his neck and was a blue baby. After a few months the mother realized that he didn't move much. Cerebral Palsy was diagnosed. The family was devastated. When he was one year old, their family yoga therapist began to massage him for an hour a day. His neck, arms, legs, spine, head and feet were massaged with mustard oil. His movements became co-ordinated and he began to crawl, stand and walk. I was introduced to him when he was about 6 years old. He walked with his heels raised, the coordination of his hands were not perfect. He had a squint and could not speak coherently.

I began to treat his neck and massaged his legs and arms. The yoga master's treatment combined with mine began to show better results .He could run and speak better. He went to a normal school. The yoga master used his exercise techniques for coordination and movement while I focused mainly on my massage technique. This went on for several years. I bonded with the boy very well and he used to ask me a lot of questions. I left India but did see him occasionally to meet him during my trips there. Years later, I met him in his office. He was the managing director of a large company. I was so pleased for him.

I always believed in one simple logic: If lack of blood flow to the brain is the primary cause of such disability, then improved circulation to the brain, at an early stage will cure it or reinstate some basic functions.

Most children that I saw were in late stage and they made some recovery with physiotherapy. It was too late for any substantial improvements of their condition. Those who came early showed very good results.

* * * * *

A friend of mine, Enzo Manes, operates a well-organized camp for sick children with a charity called 'Hole in the Wall' started by Paul Newman. It's called Dynamo camp and is based in Enzo's copper company's (KME) estate in northern Tuscany, Italy. Sick children go there for a highly enjoyable break where they can play, swim, sing, dance and have fun. The volunteers look after such children and so parents get a break.

I did a two-day seminar for parents of disabled children, teaching parents my technique of improving blood flow to the brain. The children with cerebral palsies showed noticeable improvements. The spasticity improved, the drooling became less and they were a lot calmer. One child who used to get several epileptic fits a day, was having one every few days. Then had one attack a month and is now off medication.

Dynamo camp was not meant to be a treatment center and it is not licensed for that. My over enthusiasm to treat those disabled children has caused a dilemma. The parents want to learn more of the technique but there are logistical problems. There are other children with cancer, leukemia, genetic disorders and disabled or neurologically affected children cannot be singled out .A wealthy Russian friend of mine, Georgy Bedjamov has promised to help such children. He already supports disabled children in Russia.

11.2 Epilepsy

One of the main causes of epilepsy is trauma to the brain. Another cause is brain tumor. The normal treatment for such episodes or fits is drugs that suppress the electrical activity of the brain. The brain generates electrical charge, rather like the rain clouds, which are then sent down to the rest of the body through nerves to cause involuntary contractions of muscles in quick succession, almost like lightening. This is called Grand Mal seizures. Another type Petit Mal, causes absentia or the person affected momentarily become blank loosing all communication with the outside world. It's like someone switching off completely for a few seconds.

I have successfully treated several children and a few adults with epilepsy. The results are so noticeable that some physicians contacted me to find out exactly how this treatment worked. I could only explain using logic but Evidence-Based Medicine needs scientific proof.

* * * * *

An Asian boy of four was brought in to see me. The boy had 8-12 seizures a day and was put on anti-epileptic drugs. Doctors increased the dose to the maximum but even that didn't stop the seizures. I taught the parents how to do the treatment and the child was brought in to see one of my assistants every week. After just a few treatments, the fits stopped. He is now over eight years old and has not had any more seizures. The doctors think they have hit the right level of drugs and are reluctant to reduce the dose.

* * * * *

When I was doing my seminar at The Dynamo Club in Tuscany, a little boy of two was brought to me. The parents were very distraught as the child had several seizures an hour. Drugs did not help. He was a forceps delivery and was a blue baby at birth. I explained my technique on a one to one consultation. I showed how the neck and head massage had to be done.

The parents did this therapy twice a day. After 3 weeks the results were astonishing as the boy had only a couple episodes a day. At the open day at The Dynamo Camp, this boy's success story was mentioned in a gathering of over a thousand parents, donors and volunteers. By then the boy had the seizures only a few times a month. I hope to see the child again after a year to assess his condition. I am confident that he like the others will show remarkable results.

* * * * *

There was the case of an Arab child, 5 years of age who started getting fits quite suddenly. He was brought to London and had every possible test done but nothing concrete showed up. I examined him and asked if he played exciting video games with flashing lights. The answer was `yes'. The parents were reluctant to start any treatment as they were seeking some homeopathic or herbal solution in place of chemical drugs. I managed to coax them to have a few sessions and also taught their maid how to do the treatment. Within a few days the fits stopped. They threw away all the video games.

The son of a well-known Golfer had upto 5 fits in an hour. His birth was difficult as he came out with the Occiput first. His illness caused great tension and the father's performance was affected .As he was a friend , he allowed his son to be treated by me. After two months of treatment the seizures stopped. Sadly he has some other emotional problems . The family moved abroad and I could not continue with his treatment.

11.3 Problems with the Immune System

The pituitary-hypothalamus complex must definitely give command to control the immune system. Exactly how that is done is not known but there are definite and strong indications that some sort of coordination has to take place. Since scientists do not know why the fat bone marrow suddenly produces white blood cells (our lymphocytes) in response to an invasion by bacteria in the body, they regard this as a 'spontaneous' reaction. It simply can't be so. There has to be a higher command from the brain, which has the information of everything that goes on in the body. The white blood cells behave as if they are 'individual' soldiers carrying out the job of ridding the body of the invading bacteria, virus, fungi, pollen, allergens, chemicals etc. Even soldiers need some High Command to function. The number of white blood cells, what type and where they should be directed depends not only on the chemicals the invasion site generates but also on the analysis and the subsequent instructions from the pituitary-hypothalamic complex.

* * * * *

A three-year-old girl was brought to me with a very complicated history. She was born with a terratoma in the lungs. Terratoma is not a tumor but an actual foetus that doesn't grow outside the body as twin but in one of the organs. Its like having a brother or sister growing inside you and not alongside, sharing the mother's blood. In this case the foetus stopped developing when it reached a tennis ball size. It is called a 'tumor' because it grows inside the body. In a vast majority of cases, this additional foetus / twin does not differentiate much into organs and ultimately stops growing. It then becomes a 'tumour' in the body like a benign mass.

This girl was on antibiotics ever since she was born. She coughed and was breathless all the time. Her immune system was so poor that she harboured an infection, almost continuously, in the lungs. The chances of her survival were poor.

Professor Buteyko, the well-known Russian breathing expert was my guest and staying in the flat above the clinic. He cured asthma, allergies, blood pressure etc with his retention-breath technique. It did originate in the principles of yoga but the Professor studied it for years and developed it to make it more applicable.

The mother came to see Professor Buteyko but when I saw her, I said I would like to treat her. Since the child was too young, she couldn't be trained to do complicated breathing exercises

I changed her diet and organized a daily massage using my technique .She saw me about twice a week initially for the neck and head treatment. Within weeks she started feeling better. With the cooperation of her Pediatrician I got her off antibiotics. She improved dramatically. If she had the slightest cold, she would be brought to me and I would give her my sinus oil, extra boost of vitamins and do my trademark neck massage. Within a couple of days she would recover.

As soon as her infection was better, she, like the hundreds of children that I have treated, began to grow. The growth hormone is secreted by the pituitary gland so its stimulation can make children grow. As this child grew the terratoma became relatively smaller and stopped occupying a proportionately large part of the lungs. Soon it became insignificant and an inert mass. Today she is a beautiful girl, rides horses and lives a normal life. She was my favourite patient at the time and I grew very fond of her.

I really can't recall how many young children I have been able to help with their immune systems. It will certainly run into hundreds. Children born with forceps or ventouse and with various forms of birth injuries, have in as many as 90% of cases had some complications or the other. The most common one amongst them is frequent colds and coughs. These children will catch infections very easily. If they are put on antibiotics (which have no effect on viruses anyway), their immune system is further run down. They get allergies like eczema , asthma etc. I teach parents to massage such children daily for three months or so until they are better.

11.4 Eczema and Asthma

Hektor barely 10 weeks old was brought to me with extensive exudative (oozing) eczema. The mother Mimi hardly had any milk and the baby was fed with formula milk from day one. The birth of the baby was also complicated. That was the youngest baby I had seen with such widespread eczema.

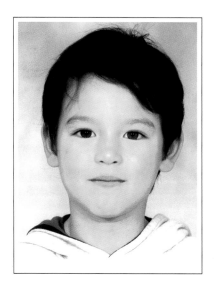

I explained to the mother that I needed her full cooperation in the baby's diet and treatment. I taught her how to massage the neck, spine and also general areas like the arms and legs. At first she was nervous but then got used to giving him massage every night before bed. The baby was quiet at first but the itchiness and rash continued. I introduced solid organic food at 5 months using pureed fresh food. The massage continued daily. Finally at 6 months or so, the eczema started getting better and the patches were restricted to the hands, elbows, and ankles. The treatment continued and in about 18 months he was clear of eczema. I used homeopathic remedies for any colds or coughs he had and never used antibiotics. I had an understanding with the mother that if the child had any signs of an ongoing infection like running nose, sneezing slight fever etc she would bring him to me as soon as possible. I would use massage, vitamin drops, my sinus oil drops for the nose and diet (chicken stock or marrow-bone soup, carrot and apple juice etc) to cure him. It worked every time.

* * * * *

 In 1994 or so, I had collected my patient's notes (some 25 of them), and with the help of my friend Dr. Michael Gormley, a well- known GP, went to see Dr. Andrew Bush, a consultant at The Royal Brompton Hospital in London. I explained that by using a simple but nourishing diet and massage, I was able to treat eczema and asthma in children. He was fascinated with the idea. Breathing exercises were also used for asthma patients.

Further communication was started and we spoke about setting up a trial using my technique.

After a few weeks, I got a disappointing letter from Dr Bush as the Ethical Committee refused to accept the proposal to carry out this trial. The reason given was quite unspecific. They said the diet and massage weren't a treatment and so could not be used for clinical trial. How strange!

* * * * *

Years later I was called by a Russian mother to see her daughter at The Royal Brompton Hospital. She begged me to see her even though she was admitted in the intensive care unit. I saw the notes and immediately took up the case. The 2 year old was a patient of Professor Andrew Bush.

The child had been born with terratoma in the liver and so the organ was very large and pushed the diaphragm up. This caused constant breathlessness. She had a tracheostomy (a tube in her bronchus to aid breathing). She was on antibiotics from the day she was born. A tube fed her.

I recommended the marrowbone soup, vitamins and mineral drops and taught the mother to do the neck massage. I sent a colleague to do the treatment in the hospital once a week.

After two months, her breathing was stable and she stopped wheezing. She was taken off antibiotics and was discharged home. The treatment continued. The little girl began to run around and became a joy for the other children. The tracheostomy was kept open as a precaution just in case she had a lung infection. She never did.

When the little girl was about 5 years old, the doctors decided to remove the terratoma from the liver. It was a risky surgery that was to last several hours. The parents agreed, as they wanted their lovely daughter to lead a normal life.

I got a call late on the day of the surgery from the mother to say that her daughter died on the operation table. I was deeply saddened. In life, sometimes you fail. She was a beautiful little child.

11.5 Growth

Almost all of the children I have treated using my technique have had a spurt of growth. The pituitary gland produces growth hormone and so this happens. In fact I tell the parents who do the treatment to their children that as soon as they notice growth in their children, they should know that the treatment is working. It is a telltale sign of the pituitary- hypothalamic area being stimulated.

I often wonder why so many children are experiencing rapid growth nowadays. The population in general is taller in developed countries than in the past. It must either be something in the diet that is stimulating, the growth hormone, or that the pituitary gland is functioning abnormally in response to the increased stress around the children.

11.6 Psychological or Emotional Problems

Children born with birth injuries or have trauma to the head and neck area, often have emotional problems. To begin with these children often become hyperactive. They are fidgety, break things in the house, become very demanding, often spin around a lot, show signs of autism etc. Most children with hyperactivity or Attention Deficit Disorder (ADD) had some sort of trauma at birth or shortly afterwards. This could be a co-incidence but an amazing one, if so. Neck massages started earlier do help such children.

The son of a friend was born with a forceps delivery. He grew up, as a slight chesty baby. The mother was very health conscious and so tried to feed him properly. One day at dinner I saw her son unusually hyperactive. I asked her if he had some birth trauma and she confirmed that. She also said that the teachers at the Play school where he was going were complaining about him being rough with the children. She was even called to the school a couple of times for his slightly violent behaviour. This child, like most hyperactive children ,demanded sweets all the time. This is an indication that the appetite center in the brain was not receiving enough glucose through the blood. I warned her that he could get further complications and she should start the neck massage. She went down the conventional medical way, consulting pediatricians and child psychologists. Drugs were prescribed to calm him down. Then he had his first epileptic fit and more followed. She had to go back to her country and it was too late to carry out any therapy. The boy became an autistic.

* * * * *

I have questioned many young ladies with eating disorders. Strangely enough most of them had either birth traumas or some fall or accident in childhood. Their necks are usually very stiff and regular neck massages coupled with psychological therapies help them a lot.

In bulimics, I notice that there is a marked improvement with treatment of the neck. Soon after eating, some of these girls feel very nauseous and they throw up. After eating when the blood rushes to the abdomen to aid digestion, and the brain is deprived of oxygen. This probably triggers the queezy sensation and they have to rush to the toilet. Sometimes they use the fingers or toothbrush to help them with the throwing up. After my neck massages this nausea subsides and they are able to override the guilt of having eaten too much.

On my Himalayan trips at an altitude of 4000-6000 ft, I have been able to cure bulimia in three women who specifically went there for treatment. The yoga, walks and massages helped their general well being. The altitude accentuated their feel good factor as the haemoglobin level in blood elevated and the treatments, including the neck massage, created positive emotions in them. The combination of this emotional uplifting and the desire to get well again did the magic.

I can confirm that many children born with some degree of trauma at birth have emotional problems later as they grow. In the early stage of their life you may not notice much change as children are naughty or very quiet but when they reach teenage, eating disorders, depression and poor self esteem often manifest themselves. Those who do sports and enjoy general well being overcome their difficulties quite well. Those with Ali Syndrome have poor comprehension. During consultation, I often have to repeat my explanation a few times. They argue , get angry and are convinced that I don't understand their complaints. I often resort to a quick manipulation or massage of the neck to improve the blood flow. They often cry with emotions(the Limbic system becomes alert) after that. The quick rush of blood changes their perception of the world. The vision improves and there is an instant "feel good factor". After that the consultation becomes smooth and productive.

It is not easy to prove the link between emotional problems and birth injuries as easy as it is to prove the physical symptoms. One of the reasons is that emotional problems or behavioural problems cannot be easily quantified. There are a lot of people in society who need psychological help but get on with life because they themselves do not complain or see it as a problem. It's others who suffer because of their behaviour. So nobody can do anything about it unless their behaviour becomes criminal or totally unacceptable.

Nervous Disorders

12.1 Cranial Nerves

Cranial nerves are those that originate in the brain while all other nerves originate in the spinal cord.

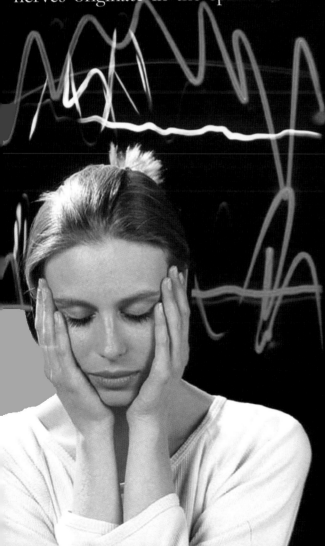

There are 12 pairs of cranial nerves that emerge from the skull or cranium. As they have direct links with the brain, circulatory deficiency to the centers or their roots (as they emerge from the brain) will cause corresponding malfunction of these nerves.

All nerves need nourishment, as they are physiologically very active. Energy requirement in the nerve and its root is very high. The nerves and their roots have very tiny capillaries called vasa nervosum (blood vessels of the nerves). As cranial nerves emerge directly out of the brain, the blood vessels that generally feed them, originate from the branches of the vertebro-basilar arteries or their branches that form the circle of Willis that encircle the pituitary gland.

In post-trauma, as in whiplash injury, a lot of people suffer from visionary problems like partial loss of vision, blurred vision, double vision etc, tinnitus, facial pain, loss of sense of smell, loss of taste etc. These symptoms may not appear immediately after the accident. They may take several months to appear. It is for this delayed effect, that there is often a big dispute between the insurance companies and the claimants. Hopefully, this book will clear some serious misunderstanding on this matter. I may not be popular with the Insurance Companies.

12.2 Trigeminal Neuralgia

This is often called 'Tic Dolores' or episodic painful attacks. If you consider all the pains in the body, then kidney stones will take the number one position. After that migraine and trigeminal neuralgia will jointly take the next position. It is so painful that one should not wish this pain or your worst enemy. During an attack, one half side of the face will hurt intensely. There are three roots of the fifth cranial nerve; one to the forehead (above the eye brow) and temple area, one to the cheek, and the lower branch or root to the lower jaw. Sometimes all these hurt together and that is hell. Sometimes, one or the other root is involved. I remember a Sikh gentleman had it in the lower branch. So severe was the pain that he used to vigorously rub his lower jaw so much that his beard on that side was uprooted. For a Sikh, keeping a beard is an essential part of his religion.

* * * * *

A 75-year lady from Melbourne was house-bound for 8 years because of the facial pain due to neuralgia of the top and middle branch of the Trigeminal nerve. She had a face-lift and the skin was straightened with a cut to the front of the ear. That's where the trigeminal nerve emerges out of the cranium. The nerve got inflamed due to a trauma caused during surgery or perhaps get compressed by the formation of scar tissue.

Her pain was so severe that the slightest touch would trigger off the attack. She couldn't wash her face or hair because of this. As a woman, she couldn't apply cream or care for her face. It was hell. She never went out, as she felt unclean. She slept on one side only. She avoided draught on her face as even this would trigger the attack. She used a scarf on her face all the time.

She heard of me from a mutual friend. We spoke and I promised to do my best. Without seeing her in person, it was difficult for me to give a prognosis. She was too afraid to fly as she was petrified of aircraft's air conditioning.

After several months of postponement, she finally flew to London with her 85-year old partner. She had severe pain and terrible jet lag when she arrived. Finally after two days she came to see me in the clinic. She was nervous as she thought I would touch or massage the area that was affected. She was totally surprised when I treated her neck. She was greatly relieved.

After only 5 sessions, the pain disappeared. She was completely euphoric. She went to the hairdressers had facials and even dyed her hair for the first time in 8 years. She began to smile again, even smiling could trigger the attack in the past. We had fun times together. She bought toys for my sons and showered us with gifts .It changed her entire life.

* * * * *

In 1996, I was invited to speak at a conference on Trigeminal Neuralgia where dentists discussed various causes of the disease. Most seem to think that the artery (a branch of the vertebro-basilar artery) that feeds the trigeminal nerve makes a loop around it and mechanically scratches or irritates it, causing severe pain. In 30% of cases, scans show that this artery does have anomalies or loops. My argument was: what happens in the other 70% of cases? I made a confident and convincing presentation, explaining my stand on the reduced blood supply to the trigeminal nerve, as the main cause. The dentists were impressed and found the logical explanation very convincing. They were not so appreciative when I added that during excessive dental work, the neck is often traumatized and the vertebrae get disaligned and this often causes trigeminal neuralgia. I should have been more diplomatic as they have to do whatever they have to do. They are not to blame. They need to operate with special chairs or with patients lying down flat or under general anaesthesia in complicated cases.

* * * * *

Treatment of trigeminal neuralgia with my technique is a dramatic proof of the link between cause and effect. Many patients call this 'magical treatment' or 'incredible healing' as my touch or massage (in the appropriate area) cures the condition quickly. They think I have healed them with my hands. I am glad every time I successfully alleviate such severe pain in patients after years of suffering. No material thing in the world can substitute for that feeling. I am proud of my profession.

* * * * *

A Spanish aristocrat lady came to see me in Madrid. She was petrified of touching her face . For six years life was hell because of one-sided facial pain, which was constant. On questioning it seemed she had had some accidents. I treated her neck and after the first session she felt relief. I gave her a few sessions and she was pain free. She told other patients with Trigeminal Neuralgia to see me. She couldn't believe it.

Normally, such patients would be prescribed strong painkillers or anti epileptic drugs as the symptoms come in episodes.

12.3 Burning Tongue and Mouth Syndrome

Many people experience intolerable burning sensation on one half of the tongue. Some experience burning sensation on one half of the palate. Both these conditions are episodic or manifest themselves in attacks of extreme discomfort. The sufferers can't eat, chew or swallow. They feel as if they have a hot charcoal in the mouth.

I have treated several cases of these two conditions, using my technique.

12.4 Loss of Taste and Smell

After whiplash injuries, head injuries and other traumas many people experience loss of taste or smell. Since these sensory functions are not lost immediately after the trauma but manifest themselves months later, it is difficult to link the symptoms to the cause. Cranial nerves control taste and smell so, as in the case of others mentioned above, there must also be a link.

I must confess that my treatments in this area haven't always been successful. These are highly sensitive and delicate nerves. Improving blood flow after a long gap (since the trauma) doesn't always help. One doesn't know the damage until much later so treatments cannot be applied in time. No one seeks advice before the symptom appears. I have a few cases where treatment was applied within weeks of the loss of sense of smell .They got rid of the sensation very quickly.

A young man in his late twenties tripped and fell on his face. Immediately the sense of smell was lost. A few months later he could regularly smell coffee. I gave him a session of neck therapy and gave him some aroma therapy oil to smell. He could smell again. I told him to continue with neck massage with a Sports Injury Therapist.

Its in 'my own experience' that there is a link between head and neck trauma and disturbance in taste or smell. When I was a teenager I joined the boxing group in my boarding school in class 8. I was skinny and tall, so my sports teacher said that my long hands and lightweight could give me an advantage. I trained to box, jogging in the morning and punching bags. My dreams fell apart, when my opponent gave me some good punches in the face, during a practice round. That evening I began to smell raw egg! About two days later I lost my sense of smell. I went to the school nurse who told me rest. After a week or so my sense of smell came back. There is the link.

12.5 Tinnitus

Tinnitus is one of the most common neurological conditions in people above 40 years of age. One hears a sound (buzzing, whistling,) continuously even though there is no external source of this sound. It is annoying, especially when it is loud. If one fails to ignore it then this dominant sound can cause extreme irritability. It is said that Van Gough cut his ear off because he got fed up of his tinnitus.

Most of those who come to see me within three months of the onset of this symptom show good results with my treatment. In the chronic stage the improvement is negligible.

The hearing nerve (auditory nerve) must get adequate blood supply for it to function optimally. Reduced blood supply can cause high pitch noise. Substantial loss of blood supply to the auditory nerve can cause deafness.

Loud music or explosion can cause tinnitus as well. This is not connected to problems in the neck. The sudden impulse of the sound waves causes some damage to the inner ear where sensitive nerve endings pick up the sound. Many war veterans who have been very close to the scene of loud explosions have tinnitus.

Tinnitus is a common symptom in people after whiplash injuries. As with other symptoms, they appear later.

12. Loss of Vision

The optic nerve that is responsible for vision is located close to the pituitary gland. The same circle of arteries that feed it, also supply nutrition to the Optic nerves. Of all the sensory functions, vision is most sensitive or powerful. Whether your hearing, taste and smell has improved or deteriorated slightly is hard to tell, but if your vision has changed you will notice it immediately. Most people who have neck manipulation and almost everyone who has my treatment of the neck, report sudden and amazing brightness in the eyes. They say that they can see well. As more blood flows into the Optic nerve, the vision improves. It may not be a permanent thing because it will take a few sessions to achieve that.

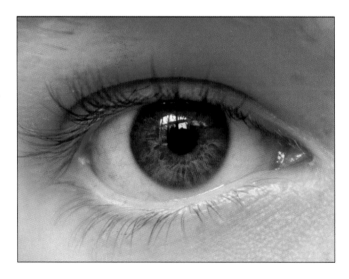

A 747 pilot of Cathay Pacific was rock climbing in Hong Kong. He fell and hit his head on the rock. He was treated in the hospital where he regained consciousness. He had headaches, dizziness, fatigue, and partial loss of field vision on one side. It was this last symptom which scared him the most. As a pilot he had to have perfect vision. He was extremely worried. He came to see me in my clinic in Hong Kong. I began to treat his neck and gave him some yogic eye exercises. His vision began to improve after a few sessions. He later joined me on my Himalayan Health Trip, where the effect of altitude helped to further improve the blood supply to the nerve, massage was done regularly. The combined effort of raised haemoglobin after acclimatization and treatment with my technique helped him tremendously.

He went back for an eye test, had a few extra training at the simulator and went back to flying again.

* * * * *

Some 20 years ago, a close friend of mine, Frank Chapman, lost vision on one-half of the field in one eye, after a fall. This condition is called Hemiopnia. He was extremely worried as driving, reading, working became very difficult. He went to the best doctors in London and steroids were prescribed. I put him off coffee and excess salt, showed him the yogic eye exercises and began to treat his neck area. After only a few sessions his eyesight improved and the field of vision was restored to normal.

* * * * *

An 80 year old was diagnosed with Macular degeneration. With this condition your vision becomes weaker and you may loose your central vision. It is linked to the degeneration of the optic disc in the back of the eye. In short, degeneration of the optic nerve causes the loss of vision .It is considered to be an incurable condition and usually blindness follows.

I began to treat her and gave her some exercises for the eyes and neck. The vision stabilized after the initial improvement and she sees a lot better. Luckily, someone close to both her and me arranged the appointment when the diagnosis was just established.

* * * * *

A gamekeeper came to see me for partial loss of vision. He had to retire because of his eye condition. I asked him if he had any head or neck injury. Initially he said he didn't. Midway through my treatment he said he had fallen off a horse and hit his head on a rock. Shortly after that his vision started to deteriorate. The link was established. He had some treatments and I showed his wife how to massage the neck. He also did the eye exercises, which is my standard treatment for all eye problems. His vision was restored to normal.

* * * * *

The owner of a large Estate in Scotland had loss of vision in one eye. He came to see me after recommendation from a friend. I asked him about some accidents prior to the onset of this symptom. He said he had no accident or trauma ever. He came back the following day and said he recalled an incident prior to the visionary problems. He was carrying the gun over his shoulders and had both his arms on either side of the gun. As he walked, he felt dizzy and slightly sick. He sat down to rest. He felt better but a few days later his vision started to deteriorate. He was quite amazed at the link between the neck trauma and his symptom. He noticed an improvement after a few treatments.

* * * * *

Very often people can't recall accidents. After the treatment the improved blood flow stimulates the memory center in the limbic system of the brain and patients are able to recall better.

People who are about to faint see darkness but if they are helped immediately to lie horizontally, the vision is restored as blood flows into the retina and optic nerve.

12.7 Pituitary Hypothalamic Malfunction

Both the pituitary gland and the hypothalamus get blood supply from a ring of arteries called 'The Circle of Willis', a major branch of the vertebro-basilar arteries. I have mentioned various complications in different sections of the book but in this chapter I will deal with specific conditions.

12.7.1 Thyroid Malfunction

The thyroid glands are located in front of the neck. Iodine absorbed in the gut is transported to the thyroid glands where the cells manufacture and release the thyroid hormones. There are two types of thyroid hormones: T3 containing 3 molecules and T4 containing 4 molecules of iodine. Both the synthesis and secretion of T3 and T4 are controlled by the pituitary hormone called the thyroid-stimulating hormone (TSH). TSH increases production and release of T3 and T4 from the thyroid which exert negative feedback on TSH production i.e if T3 and T4 appear in blood in ample quantity the production of TSH will slow down(negative feedback) .   So if the body needs more T3 or T4 the hypothalamus, sensing the deficiency, will signal the pituitary gland to secrete TSH, kick start the manufacturing process and release it. Thus there is a strong link between the headquarters and the factory.

Functions of thyroid hormones (T3 and T4) are quite simple. These hormones penetrate all cells of the body and help to generate energy. They help to burn glucose inside the cell structures called mitochondria with the help of oxygen to do that. So they facilitate "burning" of glucose or fuel and thus increase the metabolic rate. The more glucose you burn the more energy you get. If T3 and T4 secretion is less, the metabolic rate drops, the body slows down. The excess glucose, which is available through digestion, in any case, will then get deposited as fat. Thus malfunction of thyroid gland will slow down production of T3 and T4, which in turn will increase in the release of TSH from the Pituitary gland. So when someone has low thyroid it means the metabolic rate is slow. Patients will experience weight gain, cold hands and feet, feel hot and cold, hair loss, low blood pressure, depression, dry skin, constipation and chronic fatigue. With slow metabolism one feels very sluggish. The normal solution is to prescribe Thyroxine, the synthetic thyroid hormone to help with this situation. This may help with fatigue, low blood pressure, abnormal heat sensation etc but does not change the weight. That is because the fat deposited all over the body is mostly hormonal white cellulite fat and not dietary yellow fat. People did not eat extra to gain this weight it is just that there was a fault in the brain, which resulted in the reduction of the metabolic rate.

There are other causes of thyroid malfunction. Lack of iodine in diet causes poor synthesis of T3 and T4. So when there is a demand of these hormones, the TSH is secreted all right but the lack of raw material (iodine) prevents production or synthesis. The TSH makes the gland swell up with extra cells but the T3 and T4 secretion is poor. The large swelling of thyroid gland is called goiter.

There is another common type of thyroid malfunction called Hashimoto's disease. This is when the immune system gets angry and, as with rheumatoid arthritis, Lupus etc, begins to attack the body's own tissue. That is why it is called autoimmune disease. In this case the thyroid tissue is inactivated or destroyed by the angry antibodies and no T3 and T4 can be produced. Here immuno-suppressing drugs become more useful as a damage controlling measure.

Excessive production of T4 and T3 which is a "panic state" of Pituitary-Hypothalamic region, causes decreased secretion of TSH(negative feedback) . The body begins to produce more T3 and T4 than required. This causes muscular tension, increased metabolism, flushing, excessive body heat, increased heart rate, panic attacks, anxiety, restlessness, mood swings, excessive sweating and weight loss. Despite the increased activity of the thyroid the body feels totally exhausted .The person feels as if he or she has run a marathon.Thyroid condition is more common in women.

Most people who suffer from Pituitary-Hypothalamic malfunction, have a history of birth injuries, trauma, accidents, whiplashes, neck injuries etc. Thyroid malfunction is directly linked to that.

Just like Thyroxin, my treatment helps to eliminate some of the symptoms of thyroid malfunction but some symptoms like weight gain do not respond. For that I need the diet programme to show improvements. With under active thyroid, the weight gain is gradual and before a blood test one doesn't know the problem. When one discovers the problem, it is often too late as in the case of auto-immune disease, loss of smell, taste, etc long after an accident or trauma in the neck.

I have examples of cases where my treatment improved the T3 and T4 level but the weight didn't shift. Hormonal weight gain will be discussed later in the book. Such symptoms like chronic fatigue, intolerance to cold, dryness of skin, hair loss improves much faster. Patients feel generally happy but are concerned about weight

12.7.2 Disturbances in Periods (Menstruation)

The Pituitary stimulates the ovaries through the hormone Follicle stimulating hormone (FSH). This causes the maturation of the follicles that ultimately cause ovulation. Being the headquarters of the autonomous or subconscious functions of the body, the hypothalamus, together with the pituitary, controls the menstrual cycle.

* * * * *

A young lady did not have periods for over 6 months. She tried the pill but that didn't help. Her specialists told her that she was menopausal. That really depressed her. She came to see me. I asked her about any accident she may have had. She confirmed she fell down the stairs as a child, hit her head a couple of times and cut her chin in childhood.

I explained what the problem was. I changed her diet, gave her some supplements and gave her a series of neck and shoulder treatment. After two months she was ecstatic as she got her first period. She had slight irregular periods for 6 months and then they became regular.

I have numerous cases of women who came with period disturbances of various types. Some had long or frequent periods; some had very brief (2 days) and scanty periods while others had long cycles (over 35 days). The treatment that helped them was my technique of neck and shoulder massage.

12.7.3 Infertility

There are many women who, in spite of having normal periods and whose husbands / partners have perfect sperm count, fail to get pregnant. This is often called 'unexplained' infertility. These women are extremely stressed and IVF and other artificial methods of conception often fail. Every month that passes causes a lot of stress. Relatives, friends and colleagues often ask why they do not want to start a family. It's too embarrassing to accept infertility. A woman feels incomplete.

I have my own explanation for this. Stress does play an important role. The blood supply to the endometrium or innermost layer of the uterus is provided by vessels that penetrate the layer of the involuntary muscles horizontally. With stress the muscles contract and the blood vessels are compressed. The endometrium is starved of nutrients and the implanted fertilized egg fails to develop. Soon after ovulation, if a woman receives the sperms, the fertilization is almost guaranteed. Unfortunately she begins to worry 'will it happen or will it not'. This causes the uterus to contract. Ultrasonic examination after a pinprick test shows the uterus can contract involuntarily due to painful stimulus or stress.

My approach is to apply various types of therapies simultaneously to achieve the results. I change the diet so there is less intake of acid foods, alcohol, coffee, excess salt and yeast (to avoid bloating in the stomach.). I give them high protein diet. The neck treatment helps the ovulation, reduces stress and creates the 'feel good factor'. Some herbal supplements containing phytoestrogens mimic 'oestrogen therapy' and help to thicken the lining of the womb. Yoga achieves calm and relaxation. This integrated approach prepares the woman's mind and body to conceive.

I have had several successes and do have a number of pink or blue 'thank you' cards to prove that.

The Daily Mail interviewed a few ladies that had babies after my treatments. One French lady had a baby after 8 years of trying. After the first one she went on to have more without any effort but with changes of diet and some neck treatments. This article brought hundreds of infertile women to my clinic.

* * * * *

A woman in her late thirties tried for a child for 8 years. She had many tests, tried IVF, Chinese medicine, Acupuncture but nothing helped. She came to see me as a last resort. She confirmed she had an accident when she was in her twenties. She used computers a lot. I changed her diet and began to give her treatment for the neck, which was very stiff. After a couple of months, she didn't have periods. She was worried that the treatment didn't work. The periods were delayed by over six weeks. She went to her regular doctor who carried out a blood test and a scan. She was over the moon when she found that she was pregnant. She had a lovely baby girl. After three years, she tried for a second child but nothing happened. She came back to me and I recommended the same treatment. The following month she became pregnant and this time she had a son. This lady jokingly called them Dr Ali's children. From time to time I see the children for some minor ailments. I am very fond of them.

One couple that tried to have a baby for over seven years went on my trip to the Himalayas. They had regular massage, walked in the mountains, did yoga, and ate healthily and relaxed. Two months after the trip, the lady was pregnant. They went on to have two more children.

12.7.4 Hormonal Imbalances in Children

The parents brought a Sikh girl, 6 years old, to me. They were absolutely horrified that their daughter developed breasts, had pubic hair and began to spot. They went to the specialists who recommended drugs that blocked hormones, which meant she would be infertile forever.

The girl was a forceps delivery and was blue at birth. I had not treated or seen anyone with this condition. I thought I would do an experimental treatment by stimulating the pituitary by improving the blood flow to it. I gave her some diet and prescribed an Indian remedy often used to increase sperm count. It must have some mild testosterone-stimulating properties. In three months the treatment worked. All the pubic hair disappeared and there was no spotting every month. They continued the treatment for a year .The breast however did not regress. Today she is a beautiful 26 years old with full signs of femininity.

* * * * *

The grand daughter of a well-known businessman was 6 years old when the mother noticed that she was developing breasts. Additionally, she developed strong body odour . No child would go near her in school. She developed a complex as she couldn't understand. The school complained and specialists were at their wits end.

An assistant of mine began to treat her every week. At home the Nanny and the mother did some more treatment. After a few months the breasts stopped developing and the thick hair in the pubic area became thin. The body odour was less intense but was still there. She began to grow with the treatment and so the breast did not look very prominent I have not seen her in recent years.

* * * * *

Male goats have a very distinct smell. One can identify them from afar . Similarly children with severe hormonal problems have a strong body odour. I wish I had seen more cases to study the changes before, during and after treatments. In private practice people pay for their treatments and it's not easy to see them more frequently even if I want to. Some feel embarrassed to be treated free.

12.7.5 Polycystic Ovarian Syndrome

The Pituitary Hypothalamic area stimulates the development of follicles in the ovaries. The egg cells grow in these follicles. Every month, by around mid-cycle, one or the other follicle bursts and releases the egg cell. This process is called ovulation. Sometimes due to the over-activity of the Pituitary-Hypothalamic area, excess FSH (follicle stimulating hormone) is secreted. This causes one or more of the follicules to grow abnormally large. They do not have matured egg cells to release so they become cysts (bubble with liquid). Multiple cysts form polycystic ovaries.

In male and female bodies Testosterone is the principal hormone. In females, testosterone is converted in the ovaries into estrogen. Due to the presence of cysts in the ovaries, the healthy tissue is displaced and the above conversion is not possible. Thus in PCO, there is an excess of testosterone or male hormones. The periods stop or become erratic due to lack of estrogen. In PCO women get facial hair, acne and put on excess weight (cellulite fat). These are signs of excess male hormones.

I am able to diagnose by reading the telltale signs on a patient. It is an art I have developed over three decades of practice. PCO is quite an easy diagnosis for me. If there is a specific type of weight gain (fat deposit on arm, thighs, breasts, lower abdomen), facial hair develops and specific spots appear on the iris of the eye in an area known as the ovary area. Then I know it is PCO. I confirm it with a few questions like whether there were irregular periods. When did the symptoms start? Was there an accident or birth trauma?

I have seen many patients with this condition. They are usually young, in their 20's and 30's .Some were infertile because of erratic or absence of periods. Initially I suggest a diet with practically no oil or fat (as I do in my clinical spa, Castel Monastero, in Tuscany). The food is tasty because of herbs and spices but it has no oil. It is grilled, steamed, smoked or roasted without any oil. Over a period of time, due to total lack of fat in the diet, the body starts to break down its own fat. This weight loss is enhanced by an exercise programme. Amazingly, just the weight loss alone can trigger the recovery from PCO in some women.

I integrate the weight-loss programme with neck treatment (at least twice a month), phyto estrogens (Chinese Don Quai or Indian Shatavari), Homeopathic remedies (Pulsatilla where indicated) and some vitamins. In a majority of cases the treatment works. The cysts reduce in size or disappear. It may sound like a tall claim but this result has been achieved in many cases. The facial hair disappears only when everything else is rectified. In PCO, the insulin level is often raised. Many women are prescribed Metformin, an anti-diabetic drug. My integrated approach to treatment of PCO diminishes the need for this drug as soon as the weight drops.

12.7.6 Auto-Immune Diseases

This is a group of diseases that are caused by an 'angry'or overactive immune system attacking the body's own tissue. It is as if it were allergic to its own (auto) tissue and the immune system tries to destroy it. Normally, as soon as a foreign body that the body is allergic or sensitized to (dust, pollen, allergens, pollutants, and certain foods like nuts, shellfish etc) enters the system, the detective cells (lymphocytes) and other tissues secrete histamine which produces an instant reaction like sneezing, asthma, runny nose, swelling in the eyes or throat, itching etc. This means that the body is defending itself and wants to eliminate the allergen or foreign body as soon as it can.

In auto-immune diseases something strange happens. Normally, all tissues of the body are very friendly even though they have different cells carrying out different functions. All cells have the same parents (egg and sperm) and are related: no problem there. Sometimes, due to infections, inflammation or some unknown factors, some tissues are so deeply affected that their genetic structure or identity code is changed. Such tissues include joint membrane, skin, kidneys, eyes, muscles, gut lining, lining of blood vessels etc. The immune system identifies them instantly as 'traitors' or aliens. It begins to attack these tissues as it becomes really angry. That is a bizarre reaction as the body tries to destroy or reject its own tissue, as if a tissue transplant has really gone wrong.

The angry immune system becomes more intolerant and the only way physicians can stop it is by prescribing immuno-suppressants like steroids or some drugs used in cancer therapy etc. Simple anti-histamines don't work here. By suppressing the immune system you spare the affected tissues from being destroyed.

Since the Pituitary-Hypothalamic area controls all involuntary functions, I presumed that helping it to function better would in some way help to check this aggressive disease. To my great satisfaction, it worked in many cases. If patients with auto-immune disease changed their lifestyle, controlled their stress and received my specific neck treatment, there was a good chance that the disease would go into remission. I call it 'remission' because these diseases are nasty and with more stress and bad lifestyle, they can return with a vengeance.

12.7.7 Chilblains and Reynaud's Syndrome

An example of just how diverse problems arising from the neck can be was illustrated by the case of the principal of a leading girl's school in Delhi who suffered from chilblains, even in the summer. Her toes would ulcerate and become purple. She couldn't wear shoes and had difficulty in walking. She had a weak build and ate very little. She wore woolen socks, dipped her feet in saline water, used a hot water bottle under her feet at bedtime and dressed the ulcers when they appeared.

Frankly speaking, I didn't understand what was going on. I recommended a general treatment of diet, simple yoga, some supplements and weekly neck treatment. To my great relief she began to respond. She had comfortable summers and had fewer problems in the winters. I was in touch with her for a several years and she was quite pleased with the results.

* * * * *

A leading designer in London had Reynaud's syndrome. Her hands would go white from the wrists downwards every time she washed her hands in cold water. It looked as if she wore white gloves. The cold water would cause the arteries in the hands to constrict such that there would be a total shut down of blood flow. The hands would be ice cold and painful as if she was holding ice. It was embarrassing too as those who were near would be horrified to see 'white' hands. A mutual friend sent her to see me. I explained what was happening and because it was freshly diagnosed there was a good chance that it would heal. She followed the treatment religiously and after washing her hands she would practice my special breathing. I asked her to hold her breath for 10 seconds, take in only half a breath and hold it for 10 seconds. This way she was starving her body of oxygen. Effectively speaking she was taking 3-4 breaths in a minute instead of the 18 or so that we normally take. This causes raised carbon dioxide in blood, alarming the

Hypothalamus of an eminent danger of oxygen deprivation. The hypothalamus would send messages to the arteries in the hands to dilate instantly. This counteracted the effect of the Reynaud's syndrome. She was thrilled that this breathing technique worked. She came for neck treatments every week for 3 months. She never had the attack again and began to feel overall quite well.

12.7.8 Rheumatoid Arthritis

This chronic inflammatory disease attacks both smaller and larger joints of the body. There is swelling, pain, restricted movement and heat in the joints. Nowadays, doctors go straight for steroids and immuno-suppressants to calm down the symptoms.

Cecile a friend who was diagnosed with Rheumatoid Arthritis was totally distraught. She read up on the disease and her symptoms were unbearable. The early morning stiffness and the pain were very uncomfortable. She was also very reluctant to take those heavy drugs.

At the first meeting, I told her that if she did what I suggested, the chances were that she would go into a long remission. She agreed to do everything I suggested. Incidentally, she had old childhood traumas but her neck was stiff due to a lot of stress for a prolonged period prior to the attack.

I changed her diet and did a 7 day course of treatment of the neck and some of the joints that were severely affected. I used my well-known Joint oil which contained a blend of mustard, sesame, clove, winter green and black cumin seed oil. She massaged her joints every night at bed time. This oil helped to take the pain and inflammation away locally.

After a week she started to feel better. She went to a local deep-tissue massage therapist and had regular treatment using my technique. After 6 months all her pain and inflammation disappeared. A blood test showed reduction of ESR, an indicator of inflammation in the body. Four years later, when I last saw her, she was totally asymptomatic. She recommended one other friend with a similar condition, and she too is making good progress. Her husband Janni was so pleased with her progress that he made a substantial donation to my Sagoor Charity Clinic in the Himalayas. A guest house was built there for foreign patients to have treatments for chronic ailments at an affordable price. This guest house now helps to fund free medicines to the 50,000 people who use it.

An elderly lady from a very well-known Aristocratic family in Florence had severe arthritis. It restricted her movement and deeply affected her life. She came to see me at The Castel Monastero near Siena. She had the neck treatment and it completely changed her life. She has treatment of the neck from time to time for her tinnitus, dizziness and fatigue.

12.7.9 Psoriasis

This is one of the most difficult skin conditions to treat. It affects the elbows, knees, scalp, face, body, soles of the feet, hands etc. Very often it is linked to stress. It is an autoimmune disease. Normal treatment involves steroid creams, immune-suppressants or anti-cancer drugs. Sometimes the sun and the sea help. People often get the skin cured in the Dead Sea or in hyper-saline water used in Thalasso-therapy. .The hyper-saline solution gives temporary relief to the skin, but the condition returns with a vengeance after a few days.

Just as with the other autoimmune diseases, the sooner the treatment is applied the better it is.

* * * * *

A man in his forties had had several accidents from motorbike to skiing traumas. He went through a difficult divorce and was extremely stressed. He started getting dry patches on the elbows and the body. The affected area would often ooze when the dry white skin would peel off. At night there would be a lot of itching. He used coal tar, steroid creams, ultra-violet radiation etc. They gave him temporary relief.

I put him on a diet of no yeast, sugar, alcohol, mushrooms citric or coffee. I prescribed my Detox powder, aiming at controlling the yeast or Candida overgrowth in the stomach. I gave him sulphur powder mixed in coconut oil which he applied on the affected areas of the skin. He had weekly neck massage.

After a few weeks the skin began to clear up. New spots would appear elsewhere but as time went by they would be smaller in size. After about 4 months his skin cleared up. He continued treatment for about 6 months and I have never seen him again.

12.7.10 Lupus

This is a debilitating autoimmune disease which attacks multiple organs like joints, kidneys, eyes, skin. Its characteristic sign is the red butterfly on the cheeks, formed by two bright red patches on both cheeks (wings) and the red nose (body).

* * * * *

A young lady who was diagnosed with Lupus came to see me within 6 months of the tests. She had had injuries from birth and car accidents. She suffered from backaches for many years and it was when her eyes were bad and her gait was affected that she went to the doctors. They diagnosed Lupus.

I began to treat her. I gave her some neck, back and eye exercises. Her eyesight improved and she could walk comfortably. The tests however did not show much change then but the treatment brought her condition into remission.

* * * * *

I wrote a column for The Mail on Sunday in the UK for almost 6 years. I used to answer reader's questions every week. Once I wrote about my treatment for Lupus. A patient who had had treatment for this condition from me and went into remission had difficulty in convincing the professor that my treatment worked. She took the article to him, thinking that he would be convinced that sometimes 'alternative' treatments worked on chronic diseases. The professor wrote to me to stop making claims and confusing patients about treatment of Lupus. There is no cure for this condition, he wrote, and it remains a life-threatening disease. What chance do I have against a professor? I cannot do research to prove it, but some 'anecdotal' evidence is there.

12.7.11 Premature Menopause

A lot of women who have had serious accidents or head injuries, often begin their menopause around 40. They may not have any symptoms like irregular periods or hot flushes, but the periods would suddenly stop. If they have had children, they do not panic much and accept it as an unfortunate thing but get on with life. Sometimes, extreme stress can bring out this condition. Once the menopause sets in, it is difficult to reverse it.

I did have a patient, however, who came to see me when her periods had stopped at 42 years, for only 6 months. This is often referred to as secondary amenorrhoea. She had had a car accident and whiplash after which she suffered from headaches and dizziness for quite sometime.

I changed her diet, put her on natural phyto-estrogens, Mexican yam, homeopathic remedies and gave her weekly neck massages. The periods came back after 3 months and became more or less regular. She had her natural menopause at 48 years.

There are numerous examples of the neck treatment being beneficial for secondary amenorrhea. Many such women have had hormone therapy but the neck treatment is the most natural way of treating them.

12.7.12 Sympathetic Nervous Dystonia

This is equivalent to the malfunction of the Sympathetic Nervous system, headquarters of which is located in the Hypothalamus. In this condition the blood vessels or capillaries lose their natural tone. They dilate in one area and constrict in the neighbouring area. This makes the skin look blotchy or marble-like. The hands and feet may be ice cold with the cheeks becoming bright in warm premises or in the sun or due to sudden emotions (blushing). The forearm may be extremely blotchy and hypersensitive to touch. They may have a small rash similar to eczema. These brown rashes or spots are often itchy. Such spots are prominent on the arm.

If one takes a fork and scratches the inner surface of the arm, just below the elbow, just once, one gets pale white lines after a minute or so instead of the expected red lines. This is called 'negative dermographism'. The pointed fork squeezes the blood vessels under the skin and they remain constricted. The normal reaction is to produce red lines as the blood vessels dilate soon after being mechanically squeezed. People may notice red patches on the skin after a hot shower or hot tub bath.

The hypothalamus loses its control over the blood vessels and that produces abnormal reaction

Some patients experience burning sensation on the forearm, feet, hands, and on the face. They may also feel the sensation of pins and needles in these areas and the legs. Many experience dull ache. These bizarre sensations prompt doctors to use strong painkillers, anti-epileptic drugs (to stop all sensations of pain) and steroids. There is very little to help patients with conventional drugs.

I have not seen many patients with this condition as it is not very common. Those that I have treated have shown remarkable results. For the pins and needles and burning sensations in the soles of feet, massaging the calves also helps. Tight calves due to cramps (caused by calcium or potassium deficiency, dehydration, lactic acid accumulation) can squeeze the nerves in that area. This can cause erratic sensory perception in the feet. But this is not Sympathetic Nervous Dystonia. This is "burning feet syndrome" common in Diabetic complication. In Diabetes , smaller blood vessels develop plaque due to sugar crystals . These block blood supply to the muscles . That causes Lactic acid accumulation and cramps in muscles of the calves.

12.7.13 Food/Skin Intolerances

As I mentioned before, the immune system is regulated by the Pituitary-Hypothalamic region. Food or skin intolerances are nothing but local reaction of the skin or gut due to unwanted particles on those surfaces.

Let's say you are allergic to soap, powder or a cream. Shortly after these chemicals come into contact with the skin, there will be a rash or an allergic reaction. Similarly if you are intolerant to chillies or fungal cheese, you will get bloating, cramps, diarrhoea etc as the gut lining will react unfavourably.

Food intolerances should not be confused with food allergies. The latter is a reaction of the entire immune system. One has to get sensitized to an allergen before the body can produce a reaction when it comes into contact again with the same substance.

Children with multiple food intolerances react much better to my treatment. They get abdominal pain and bloating from cow's milk quite often. Change to goat's milk, camel's milk, or soya milk, and the digestive problems stop. In this case it is clear that they are not lactose intolerant because milk of other animals do not cause any other problem. It is just that they are intolerant to only cow's milk and can even tolerate cow's yoghurt or cheese.

Adult food intolerance has to be treated over a period of 4 months or so. Shorter periods of treatment do not produce satisfactory results. I have a belief or hypothesis that red blood cells and immune cells (lymphocytes) replace themselves totally in 125 days or so, which is 4 months. One has to, therefore, carry out an exclusion diet and neck massages for that length of time for the new cells to recover any "old memory".

* * * * *

A woman with multiple food intolerances (aubergines, cheese, yeast, pork, pineapple and tomatoes) came to see me. With these products she would get bloating, diarrhoea, agitation in the mind and headache. She would also feel very tired .She had several accidents in childhood and was concussed after a skiing accident.

I put this lady on a diet that excluded citric fruits, alcohol, coffee, spicy food and sugars. She avoided the foodstuffs that she was intolerant to. I explained that she had to follow the diet for a minimum period of 4 months.

She did what she was told and had almost weekly massage, did yoga and took my Detox Tea for her Candida.

After 6 months she could eat some of the foodstuffs that she was initially intolerant to. I told her that she should not eat all the troublesome foodstuffs on the same day. She tried one or two on a single day and she was alright.

* * * * *

A dear friend of mine, Ken Bridgewater, who is editing this book, became intolerant to garlic. He felt terrible after eating it. In a club he belonged to they used to call him "Mr No-garlic". He avoided eating garlic for many years. Since meeting me he had gone on my India trips and had numerous sessions of massage and yoga. He didn't know that his intolerance to garlic was cured .He came to lunch one day and saw me cooking chicken with garlic. He was petrified and asked me politely if I could cook something else without garlic. I didn't as I was convinced that he was cured with so many sessions of treatment. He commented that if he was going to be ill there was no place like a doctor's house. He was amazed that he didn't get any reaction at all. He now eats garlic comfortably. Ken and his lovely wife Aileen have followed my Neck Connection theory and its amazing success for over 20 years.

12.7.14 Allergies (Hay Fever, Urticaria, Eczema)

Allergy is body's natural reaction to invading non-living particles or chemicals. For living organisms (bacteria, viruses) body's immune system develops antibodies to destroy it. Vaccinations against infectious diseases like cholera, mumps, measles, typhoid, polio, tetanus use this ability to create antibodies in the body to ward off a real infection. In the case of allergies, the process of desensitization with weaker doses of the allergen is a useful tool in reducing the reaction or even eliminating it.

Even though allergic reactions like cough, diarrhoea, hay-fever are defensive reactions, the symptoms they produce are very uncomfortable. In the case of allergies, the other reactions are watery eyes, runny nose, itchy eyes, coughs, asthma attacks (wheezing,) itchy skin, hives (urticaria) etc all of which are uncomfortable.

One day after treating a patient for headaches, she said her sinuses were completely clear and she could breathe better. I realized that the neck massage must have helped the immune system to function better by stimulating the Pituitary-Hypothalamic area.

Thus the neck treatment became an adjuvant therapy for allergies. While putting patients on a no yeast, fungus, citric, alcohol, coffee, and sugar diet, they regularly had neck treatments. If they had runny nose or allergic coughs or wheezing, sneezing etc, they would be advised to do the special breathing exercises. I give them my 'Retention Breath'. They breathe in for 6 seconds, hold breath for 6 seconds and breathe out after 6 seconds. In this way, instead of breathing 18 times in a minute (which is normal) they breathe approximately 3 times. This retention breath accumulates carbon dioxide in blood which in turn dilates blood vessels, nasal tract, bronchial tract, and eases the symptoms. This retention breath also relaxes the muscles and eases stress. This type of breathing exercises shouldn't be done by those with heart disease. Raising carbon dioxide level in blood can cause complications in heart disease.

Additionally for those with hay fever or allergic rhinitis, I recommend my Sinus oil or plain sesame oil drops for the nose. The oil forms a protective layer on the nose and prevents the particles (pollen, dust, mites, pollutant) and chemicals (sprays, perfumes, paint spirits, petrol fumes) from coming in contact with the mucosa of the nasal lining. So there is less irritation of the nasal tract and less allergic reaction.

In my experience and opinion Candida, a gut fungus, thrives on the gut wall rather like mould on bread, while doing so it sends raphae (roots) deep into the gut lining, creating micro pores. Large gut toxins which normally cannot penetrate the gut lining, find these pores useful in penetrating the gut to reach the underlying blood vessels. Thus toxins or allergens enter the blood stream. These are too large to eliminate through the kidneys so the skin and sinus are the only exit for them. The blood vessels allow these toxins to flow out of them with the blood fluid (serum) under the skin. As a result the skin swells up and looks like orange peel (hives). As the fluid contains a lot of salt, the nerve endings under the skin begin to itch violently. Thus in hives you have the sudden raised patches of skin producing unbearable itch all over the body. The only immediate solution is anti-histamine or steroid injection to stop the blood vessels from dilating and leaking fluid out.

For hives, my diet and neck treatments have been very useful for many patients with chronic hives. I also recommend my Detox Tea to curtail Candida growth in the gut, the root cause of the problem. The neck treatment is a useful tool in this condition. How exactly this happens is not clear, even to me.

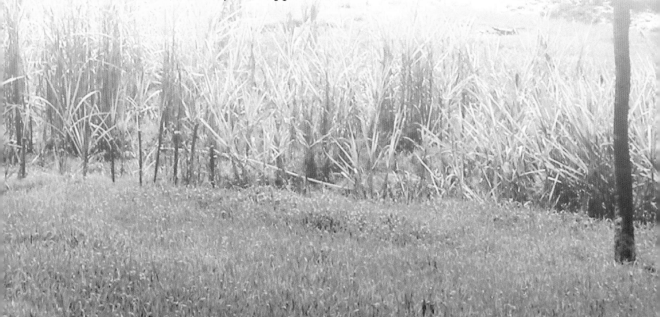

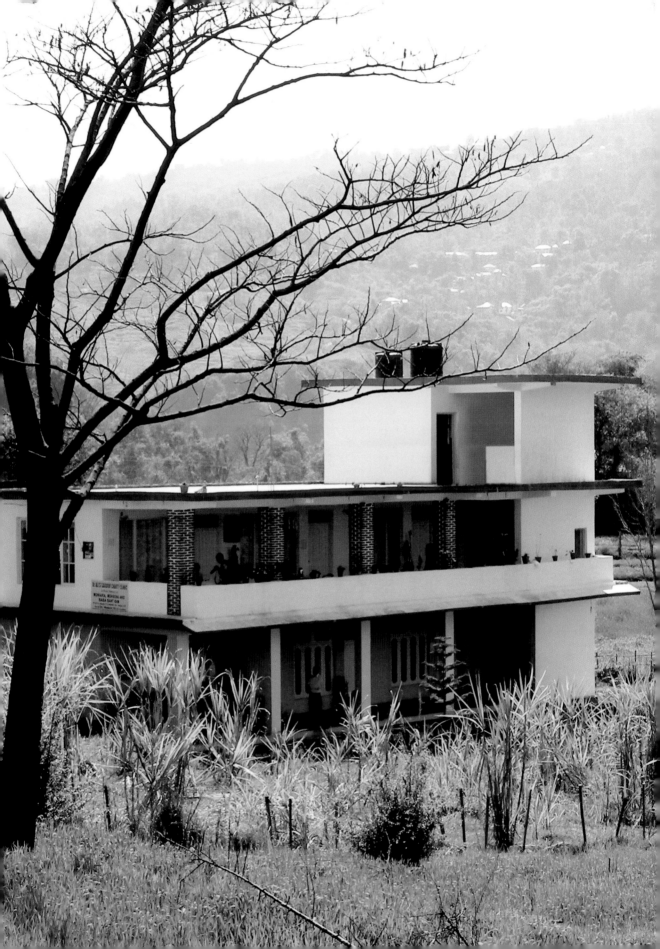

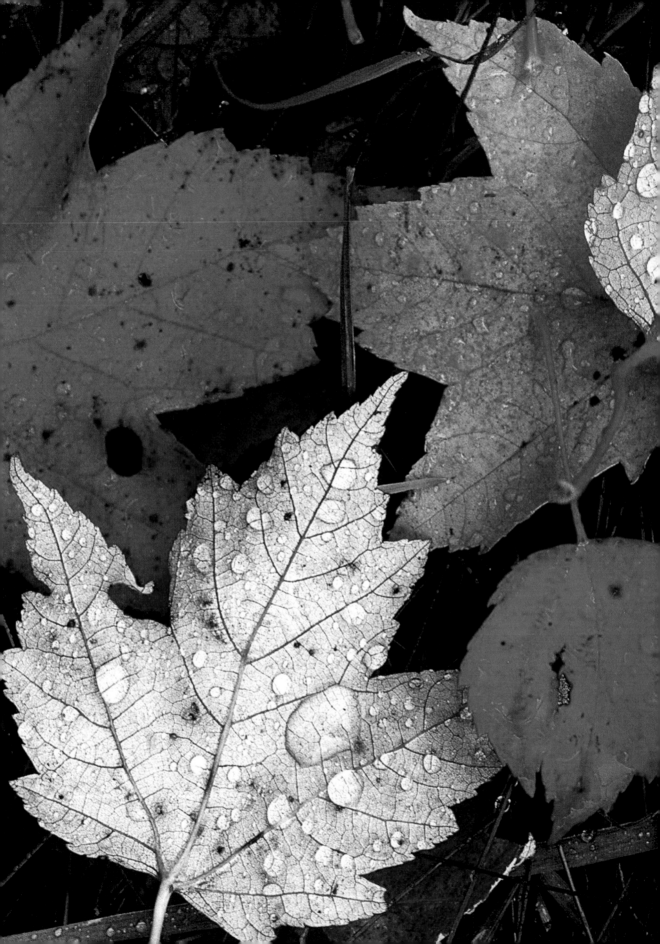

PART 3

The Solution

CHAPTER 13

Historical

The neck is a part of a whole body and should not be treated in isolation. Indeed, its treatment has to be considered in the light of all the treatments available today. Let's start at square one. To fully appreciate the present status of medicine it is necessary to have some understanding of how it developed historically. Hippocrates, who lived 2500 years ago in Greece, was regarded as the Father of Modern Medicine. His Oath is still taken by Graduating Physicians today before embarking on the practice of Medicine. If asked, no doctor now can actually say what the Hippocratic Principle of Medicine was, I am greatly influenced by his philosophy. In the 11th century another great physician Avicenna, lived in Samarkand (Uzbekistan) but travelled in the region. He used Hippocratic principles to create the foundation of what is called Unani (Unan - Eastern Greece – Ionia) Medicine. It is now practised and taught mainly in South Asia in a modified way. The original principles were largely discarded as time went by.

Hippocrates taught the following:

1. We have an innate power to maintain our health called "physis" (pronounced feesis) within us. The words "physician", "physiology", "physiotherapy", "physics" etc take their roots from it. We now understand our immune system to be part of that power.

2. The physis is a universal force present in all living beings. It analyses what goes on outside and inside our bodies, and corrects the various functions accordingly - 24 hours a day. For example if you go to a sunny place, within hours the pigmentation designed to naturally block excess ultraviolet light from causing damage to the body, will increase. You get a tan. Fins and Russians use sauna quite regularly but their skin does not darken so it's the sun's rays which, in excess, are harmful. This regulation is controlled by the physis.

3. Physis, if nurtured, can heal almost 80% of our illnesses and diseases. Emergency medicine, traumas, genetic disorders, etc constitute the other 20% and are best treated with other methods.

4. Physis can be nurtured by looking after your body and mind. This is done by eating well, exercising, relaxing, using massage, swimming, using steam or sauna, fasting periodically and sleeping adequately. In other words using common sense.

5. Natural forms of treatments (herbs, minerals, fruits, berries, etc) should be used to assist the physis to carry out its functions, normally as part of the diet.

Although a lot of time has passed since that doctrine was established, the essence of it still remains. After the death of Hippocrates, his son-in-law and others tried to establish his sayings as "dogma" or the final word in the understanding of human health and illness. There were, however, criticisms of the School of Dogmatism and so Medicine reverted to the "free thinking" mode. Christianity came and declared diseases were a form of punishment for sins. So God's influence on diseases became profound. You pray, take necessary measures provided by medicine and you'll get better. This became the general view in the West.

In the 11th century, the great Persian-Arab physician, Avicenna, revived the Hippocratic concept. He placed a lot of emphasis on the four Humours and thereby defined the constitution of individuals with a propensity to certain diseases concluding that the imbalance in the four Humours caused illness. The four factors of constitution were Sanguine, Phlegmatic, Choleric and Melancholic and the humours responsible for the diseases were Blood, Phlegm, Yellow Bile and Black Bile. A similar approach occurred independently in China.

This Humour theory was taught in Medical schools in Europe until the 16th century. Then came the Industrial Revolution and discovery of the microscope and other instruments for examination of the body. The body was viewed as consisting of separate parts and diseases were symptomatic to be treated with remedies. The concept of the body being whole was again lost in the West, although retained in the East in half the population of the world.

It was only in the 1960s in the West that alternative thinking in medicine, art, environment took root again. Alternative, Holistic and Complimentary Medicine were thus born. These looked at the entire body as one and its functions were all interlinked. The worldwide history of medicine is covered in more detail in my "Integrated Health Bible" Chapter 2.

I belong to the group of doctors who integrated conventional and traditional medicine. My maternal grandfather was a doctor and Homoeopath. I coined the phrase "Integrated Medicine" in 1982 as the future Healthcare. A doctor who has full training in conventional or Allopathic Medicine, if also specialised in Complimentary or Traditional Medical disciplines like Acupuncture, Homoeopathy, Ayurvedic, Herbal Medicine, Osteopathy, Naturopathy etc, can be called an "Integrated Medical Physician". Most such doctors will prefer one angle to another. Some doctors may choose to practice Acupuncture while others may choose Chiropractic or Herbal Medicine.

My model of diagnosis and treatment is as follows: for Diagnosis I use the Tongue, Pulse, Iridology, Eardology (examination of the ears) and General Examination. As a doctor I will look for tests, scans, x-rays whenever necessary. My treatment plan includes diet, massage, therapeutic yoga and other traditional therapy. But above all I treat the patient as a whole individual as follows. My general motto is "Treat the Diseased , not the Disease".

The Hippocratic "Regimen Therapy" is the backbone of my Lifestyle Programme which is so beautifully executed in my Clinical Spa in Tuscany. Everyone has to be on a diet , have neck and Marma Massage, do yoga and other exercises (walk in the hills , swim in the hypersaline pool, gym exercises). T he Innate Healing Power is thus aroused. This sets the 'cure in motion. Additional therapies with supplements , natural remedies, specific massages etc complete the job.
  In my London Clinic, I diagnose and recommend the Lifestyle programme and other colleagues do the specific treatments with acupuncture, herbal medicine, psychological therapies etc.

Diet

The exact dietary plan varies from region to region. People have different eating habits and the recommendations will naturally vary.

Basic Principles

The diet should exclude foods that cause damage to the body or interfere with digestion, if consumed in excess. Digestion takes place in an acid medium in the stomach (in the presence of stomach acid) and in an alkaline medium (created by bile from liver and pancreatic juice). If there is too much stomach acid then the digestion will slow down as the body has to wait for adequate alkali production in the form of Bile and Pancreatic juice before food mass can be released into the small intestine. The acid is too corrosive for the lining of the intestine

Acid helps to break down food mass and the stomach wall can then churn and make it into a pulp (chyme) so that the rest of the digestion can take place without a hitch. If we eat too fast, then the stomach has to churn more which means that digestion will require more energy. Moreover, the stomach will need to produce more juice for making the food pulp.

In the alkaline medium, finer digestion of fats, carbohydrates and proteins will take place. Soon after digestion the intestine will absorb lipids, sugars and amino acids which are the finest units of fats, carbohydrates and proteins.
The waste is eliminated by the colon. Here calcium, magnesium, water etc are absorbed before the final faecal mass is thrown out.

The Candida and Yeast Factors

In Nature there was always peaceful coexistence amongst bacteria, viruses and fungus, the three main invaders of our bodies. Then man discovered penicillin in the middle of the last century. It was a powerful fungal product and was synthesised commercially to kill off all sorts of bacteria. Although it was a useful weapon against invading bacteria, doctors began to misuse it. In the 60s they used penicillin for everything from infections to allergies. Bacteria became resistant to it. New antibiotics were synthesised and the war against bacteria began. As the organism mutated or became resistant, Medicine discovered more powerful antibiotics.

During this war between medicine and bacteria, antibiotics helped fungus and viruses to become more powerful. A fungal product (antibiotic) was used against bacteria and so fungi gained the upper hand. Viruses were too small and complicated to be affected so for a long time (before interferon was discovered) there was no real defence against them.

When I was a medical student in the 70s, bacterial dysentery, pneumonia, meningitis and other infections caused by bacteria were very common. Nowadays viral pneumonia, meningitis, gastric flu, glandular fever, viral hepatitis, cold sores, herpes, HIV, etc are more common. Similarly, fungal infections of the nails, hair roots, mouth ulcers, thrush, candidiasis, athlete's foot etc have also become very common. Thus bacteria have been replaced by viruses and fungi as the main invaders of the body.

Brewer's yeast was a common supplement for vitamin B deficiency but today the intake of yeast causes major digestion problems. Yeast in the gut, in excess, produces toxic alcohols like methanol, propanol, butanol besides ethanol which is the alcohol in beer. Uncontrolled brewing in the gut is the main cause of gas, abdominal pain, bloating and other digestive problems. It might even fail a breathalyser test.

When you consume too much yeast (bread, pizza, pitta, nan, yeast-spreads) you are also likely to get a rash and other fungal infections. The fungi in the body have their own fraternity as they help each other. Thus you can get candida (Candida Albicans) infections in the mouth, gut, vagina, around the anus (wherever there is mucus lining). The candida, like mould on bread, destroys the surface they thrive on making it "brittle" or porous. The micropores created by colonies on the gut surface, allow large toxins to penetrate through the lining and reach the network of blood vessels. An intact gut lining is non-penetrable but candida destroys that barrier. Gut toxins floating in the blood cannot be filtered out of the body through the kidneys as the molecules are too large. The only way out is through the skin and sinuses (mucus discharge). These gut toxins cause extreme fatigue and skin diseases like eczema, urticaria, dandruff, seborrhoeic dermatitis (red patches on the face), some forms of rosacea, red noses, etc. The intake of sugar helps the candida and yeast overgrowth in the gut. If one takes oral antibiotics for a prolonged period, the useful gut bacteria are destroyed and opportunistic candida infections in the gut and other surfaces develop.

Thus it is potentially dangerous to consume excess fungal products, especially if you have had recurrent thrush, bloating, mouth ulcers, athlete's foot, alopecia (hair loss in patches) on the scalp, dandruff etc.

I am against the intake of fungi, yeast, fungal products and excess sugar that feeds them. I recommend that, to build your health and to stimulate the immune system, you must avoid or at least moderate: yeast bread (soda bread, unleavened bread are OK), pizza, pitta, nan bread, beer, yeast-spread, gravy granules (instant), cheese (hard and fungal), mushrooms, Russian kvas, malt drinks, chocolates, cakes and sweets.

Basically, the fungi are parasites. They taste good and add flavour to certain preparations but they pose a risk to the body. By living off the body, in the gut, they do deprive you, as do worms and parasites, of some essential nutrients. Some mushrooms can kill you, blind you and some can potentially paralyse you. Edible fungi have their toxins too, except that their direct effect on the body is not noticeable. Look at the fungal toxin from the penicillin mould. It kills bacteria and harms us. The "weakening" of the body by penicillin toxins invites another fungus (candida) to invade our body to cause thrush, bloating, abdominal cramps, diarrhoea etc. A fungal toenail, athlete's foot, mouth ulcers, alopecia on the scalp, groin rash etc cause great discomfort and look bad on the external surfaces. We do not know the extent to which fungi damage our body and I do not know of any study on that. For example, the yeast in the gut produces a range of toxic alcohol that goes straight to the liver. What happens next over a long period of time is anyone's guess. The extreme drowsiness that follows an hour or so after a good sandwich or carbohydrate meal is a noticeable symptom.

I have also discovered that, with yeast and candida overgrowth, people get highly sensitive to white wine and champagne. Within 10 minutes of drinking these types of alcohol, you get drunk and very heavy headed. Some even get headaches and feel sick. They pass it off as "allergy" or "intolerance" to white wine. Even though all drinkable alcohols contain ethanol white wine and bubbly (the fizz helps absorption) get absorbed more quickly.

The rapid absorption of white wine or champagne lets in existing toxic gut alcohols produced by yeast into the bloodstream. The liver gets bombarded with a lot of ethanol as well as toxic alcohols, sending it into shock. It cannot metabolise them immediately so allows them to enter the main bloodstream, hitting the brain - thus the bizarre reaction. This is my hypothesis, I have not proved it. Treating the candida and yeast for a period of time, such unpleasant effects are eliminated in people and many of them have managed to enjoy these drinks again. That should logically prove my point.

If you eat mushrooms, pizza, low yeast-containing bread etc occasionally these need not be a problem. The body seems to cope with it. It's the regular and excessive use of fungal products that cause the problem.   My motto is moderation and variety in all things and nowhere is this more applicable.

There are several products you could be intolerant to in the course of your lifetime. You will know such products because you will probably get diarrhoea, bloating, gas, headaches, itchy palate or urticaria every time you eat such a product. Avoid them as far as possible. It's not worth putting your body through such discomfort or agony just for the sake of some nice taste or pleasure.

For a European Diet Plan I use a simple scheme:

Avoid, especially in excess	Reason
Yeast-products	Fungus
Cheese, mushrooms	Fungus
Orange, lemon, pineapple	Acid
White wine	Acid
Beer	Fungus
Chillis, nuts in excess	Acid
Preserved food	Acid/chemicals
Sugar, chocolates	feeds fungus
Coffee	stimulant, often disrupts digestion
Foods you are intolerant to	obviously

Additionally, I advise the following: Eat slowly. Drink water at least 45 minutes after meals so that the stomach juice is not diluted. After lunch, rest a while to allow the stomach to receive maximum energy to carry out the process of churning the food. If you have an opportunity for a siesta in the afternoon or lie down after lunch lie on your left side for 15 minutes to allow stomach juice to collect for digestion and then lie on your right as this is where the stomach has the muscles that churn your food. After dinner, walk a bit, especially if you've had a late dinner. By walking, or doing mild exercises, you stimulate the mechanical parts of the digestion, i.e. churning the food. Once you fall asleep, the body will switch off most of the digestive activities because it has to carry out repair work and rest the brain that has been active all day long.

Many patients ask me what they should eat. My experience shows that if you avoid the foodstuffs that are bad or potentially harmful to you the digestive system will cope very well. It has a great capacity to rectify the minor damage caused by foodstuffs. It is amazing how I have helped thousands with my simple dietary plan, mentioned above. For details of Nutrition and Individual ailments refer to my Nutrition Bible. It is a book that also went on to be a bestseller in the UK and I enjoyed writing it.

To aid the process of quick healing and improving digestion I recommend my favourite Detox Tea. It is a blend of herbs that are traditionally used for various types of common ailments. With a 30 year clinical experience, I know it is safe to use. Its ingredients are Chiratha, Kadu/Kutki, Amla, Neem and liquorice. Only half a teaspoon full of this herbal mixture is used. It is soaked in a cup of hot water at night and drunk on an empty stomach in the morning. It is bitter and no sweets are allowed afterwards. The residue is thrown away. Since it is used in such a small dose the chances of any side-effects are negligible. In fact, I haven't recorded a single case where someone has had any complication. The taste may cause nausea but one gets used to it after a couple of tries. Detox Tea helps to neutralise the excess acid in the stomach, prevents the growth of candida and yeast in the gut and helps the liver to secrete bile. It does lower the blood sugar level and occasionally people feel light-headed for a few minutes. Some of my Type II Diabetic patients use it regularly and are pleased with the results. It reduces excessive appetite and so helps in a gentle weight loss programme. In the Castel Monastero Spa, Detox Tea is an extremely popular drink. People hate the taste but love the benefits.

I do recommend people to eat fruits and vegetables. If possible one should have a glass of carrot, apple, root ginger, mint leaves and celery juice. This gives one the enzymes that the digestive system so often needs and it also provides the body with fresh vitamins and micro-elements.

Pomegranate and sweet lime (found in South Asia) with a distinct sweet-sour taste and a specific bitter aftertaste, are my favourites. My grandfather, a doctor-homoeopath, often spoke about these juices as elixir of health and energy. My mother, his doting daughter, learnt a lot of his favourite recipes and remedies. She says that drinking fresh coconut water from time to time aids digestion. I am sure there are fruits and berries all over the world which have a beneficial effect on digestion.

Massage

Massage is an essential part of my Healing Technique. In the Orient, massage techniques like Shiatsu (Japanese), Tuina (Chinese), Marma (Indian), Boma (Malaysian) Thai etc were more therapeutic than relaxing as they are often painful. Swedish massage uses kneading and rubbing techniques and is therefore purely relaxing. Greek and Turkish massage use pummelling, slapping, rubbing and kneading techniques. These are also therapeutic in nature.

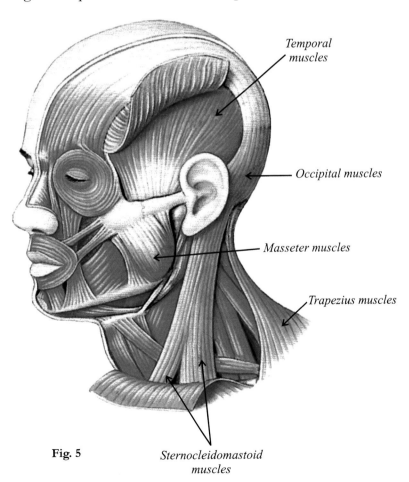

*Temporal
muscles*

Occipital muscles

Masseter muscles

Trapezius muscles

Fig. 5

*Sternocleidomastoid
muscles*

Benefits of massage

Muscles form the bulk of the body, a fact all too often neglected in the university Medical Anatomy year. Every movement in the body as well as standing and sitting, requires the participation of the muscles. Until you fall into deep sleep, the muscles are in full tone, in a partially contracted state. They need rest to replenish their energy and above all rid their bulk of lactic acid. This is a byproduct of glucose utilisation by muscles in the absence of adequate oxygen supply following excessive use and poor supply. This lactic acid can cause muscle cramp and a great fatigue in muscles. Massage gets more blood into the muscles and therefore more oxygen, which instantly converts lactic acid into carbon dioxide and water. As will be seen later, it is essential to restore relevant muscles to a relaxed and malleable state before any manipulation is attempted as otherwise any distortion can interfere with the treatment. This is especially true of the neck.

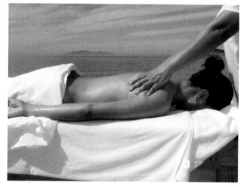

The energy molecules in the body are known as ATP (Adenosine Tri Phosphate). This is broken down by the cells to release stored energy. The muscles produce maximum amounts of ATPs. Massage is a good way of nurturing the muscles, replenishing their nutrients and keeping them toned. Exercises do similar things if they are not too strenuous (then you lose energy) and are accompanied by breathing (oxygen supply) as in Yoga and Pilates.

Massage relieves aches and pains and creates a very positive sense of "feel good factor". The skin's surface is a powerful sensory organ linked to various emotions in the body. I have tried to map it and it's quite amazing how humans and animals touch each other to generate such emotions and affection. Self touch, other than in the erogenous zones and genitalia, does not produce the same emotions. The armpit, neck, belly area, soles of feet, the area above the hips etc produce laughter (tickling sensation). The scalp induces deep relaxation and sleep. The nape of the neck and back produce "goose bumps" and sense of excitement. The areas behind the ears, lips, breasts, nipples, pubic area, the inner surface of thighs, genitalia are erogenous zones. The nostril and tickling the hair within canals of the ears and anus (orifices) cause anger.

There is constant wear and tear in the body. Massage helps to heal those, if done regularly. Repetitive Strain Injuries, as in the excessive computer use, can be prevented and treated with regular massage. In short, massage removes the lactic acid that forms 'knots' within muscles, it helps overcome fatigue, it relieves aches and pains in the joints and it activates the innate healing power of the body.

THE ALI TECHNIQUE

Having realised that the neck holds the secret to our health, well-being and illnesses, I developed a special massage, manipulative and yoga technique to treat the neck. The idea was to improve the supply of blood and cerebral spinal fluid (brain fluid) to the brain. These results are puzzling scientists.

With some caution, one can also massage the neck on one's own. It is best, however, if someone else does the massage.

When you massage the neck from the back, there is one golden rule to follow. STAY BEHIND THE EARS and you will not do any damage to the major arteries, nerves and the windpipe which are located in the front of the neck.

The neck massage can be done effectively and safely along 6 lines starting from the hairline and ending on top of the shoulder. The first pair of lines originate behind the ears. Using the thumb on one side and the four fingers on the other grab the neck. Rotate the thumb and fingers and slide them down to the top of the shoulder. You will feel hard bones. Some may stick out prominently. That is the sign of disalignment of the cervical vertebrae. Those which most often become misaligned are the third and fourth cervical vertebrae from the top (C3 and C4). These bony protrusions are often painful to touch. Massage them gently at first and then increase the pressure. These protrusions are the wings of the cervical vertebrae. Massage all of them downwards and upwards. After a few minutes they may become less sore.

Then move a couple of centimetres medially (towards the spine of the vertebrae). You will feel tight muscles of the neck. Massage upwards or downwards along the body of the muscles. Some individual muscle bundles may be sorer than others. Use your thumb on one side and four fingers on the other to massage them. Rub the muscles across as well.

Finally move towards the centre and massage the muscles that lie on either side of the axis of the spine. Some of these muscles will be sore if the patient has neck traumas or uses computers a lot. These muscles get injured during whiplash. They help to keep the chin up and therefore help to maintain posture. Massage these muscles across and downwards.

Using the thumb, massage horizontally along the hair line and above it. Here the tendons of the neck muscles attach to the occiput (skull bone). They are very sore to touch especially if your neck muscles are tight. The tendons are the extensions of muscles so they often tear and get strained with neck injuries. Massage all the tendons, till the pain eases.

Massage the areas below the ears and behind the angle of the lower jaw (mandibula). This is the area where the vertebral arteries come out of the cervical or neck canals and enter the cranium or brain. This area is covered by a thick sheath of membrane that protects the vital arteries. Massage with the thumb but with gentle pressure. This helps to improve blood flow to the brain and one often feels instantly relieved of a headache if one has one.

Massage the jaw and the temples. This eases tension and helps the skull to move freely. Ultimately this helps to improve circulation of the Cerebro Spinal Fluid that bathes the brain surface, supplying it with glucose and some dissolved oxygen.

I recommend using my Joint Support Oil which is a blend containing Mustard Oil, Clove Oil, Sesame Oil etc. You can prepare some at home using organic sesame oil (50 ml), clove oil (5 ml), mustard oil (30 ml), black cumin seed oil (Kolonji, 15 ml). The other oils used in my formula are Ayurvedic. The blending of which is my secret as its an art. Blending of alcohols , perfumes, herbs and spices , is also a creative art.

Take half a teaspoonful of the oil and rub it between the palms till it gets gently warm. This activates the ingredients and helps it to penetrate the skin to reach the muscles. The clove oil eliminates pain while the others help to relax the muscles so as to facilitate blood supply and subsequent removal of lactic acid. This reduces the inflammation of muscles.

You must remember that these muscles help to hold your head up vertically to maintain the posture. The bones of the vertebrae, skull, and shoulder just provide the surfaces to which the muscles are attached. When you fall asleep in a car or train, your head drops in all sorts of directions as the muscles lose power. The cervical spine cannot hold your head up. The head is the single heaviest organ in the body followed by the liver. It rests on a pair of pivotal joints on the top of the first vertebra of the neck. Almost 2/3 of the head lies in front of these joints and 1/3 behind, thus it is front heavy. The front part has the bulk of the brain, facial bones, eyes, tongue, teeth etc. So, like in a seesaw, the front part of the head would naturally tilt forward, but thanks to the neck muscles the chin is kept up. If we are up and about for 16 hours a day, the neck muscles work continuously during that period. By the end of the day they become stiff and quite sore from the lactic acid. Unless we massage them (passive) or exercise them (active), they would add to the problems of the neck. The joints would be stiffer and the discs would degenerate, shrinking the length of the neck. That would reduce blood flow to the brain and cause trouble.

Massaging the shoulder is also very important. The Trapezius muscle which starts at the occiput and spreads laterally to the shoulder and down to the upper spine is shaped like a rhombus with four sides. This muscle helps to support the head and keeps the chin up. One has to massage the muscles on its four sides. Thus the shoulder and upper back should also be included in the massage technique performed by a partner or therapist. He or she should try to move the head to the right and left in the supine (lying back) position. If possible, the therapist should use a towel to grip the occiput (back of the skull) and pull the head away from the body with a mild traction. One should breathe deeply while this procedure is carried out. This stretches the neck.

I have my own manipulation technique which can only be taught to medically qualified practitioners or osteopaths and chiropractors. I do not do vigorous manipulations of the neck or adjustments of the misaligned vertebrae. Some therapists do just that and do not prepare the muscles of the neck and shoulder. I know of some therapists, claiming to be qualified osteopaths or chiropractors, who just manipulate the neck. In some cases they will have several patients lying on the couches. They'll spend a few minutes adjusting the neck vertebrae, and discharging them one by one. Once finished a new batch of patients are invited for the same treatment. Patients feel good instantly but have to return to the therapist, again and again. In fact, they need repeated adjustment. It becomes a habit and is an expensive experience.   The best therapists, spend five years in college just like a medical doctor, will give the same advice I have above to tune the muscles for the treatment before manipulation is attempted and prescribe follow-up exercises.

As I mentioned earlier, the joints of the vertebrae dislocate or are misaligned or subluxated.   In the vast majority of cases, it is the muscles which create the torsion or "pull" that is responsible for putting the joints "out". Take the example of the whiplash, the movement of the neck, first forward, and then backward, traumatises the joints and dislocates them. The muscles in the cervical spine tighten up as a result of this. The therapist should work on such tight muscles and then gently adjust the joints. The results are more permanent.

Some people habitually "click" their own neck. They adjust their neck several times a day and feel good about it. The joints dislocate within a few hours, and need readjustment. One has to work on the ligaments of these vulnerable places to make sure they become firm and do not allow them to dislocate so easily. In my opinion, the more you manipulate the neck the more there is a need to do this.

Ask your osteopath or chiropractor to massage the various muscles of the neck and back. Tell them also to work on the ligaments of the facet joints. After that they need to manipulate whenever there is a subluxation of these joints. They may not like to be told what to do but you must be polite and request them to do so.

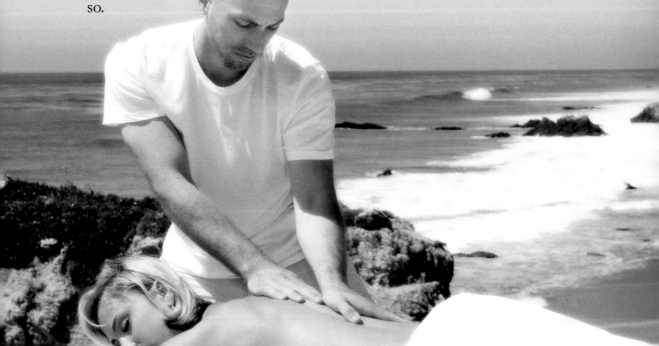

Therapeutic Yoga

Although yoga is relatively new to the West, it has a long and venerable tradition in the East. It is thought to date back to at least 3000 BC and has been practised in India to promote physical and spiritual health for millennia.

Yoga was popularised in the West during the 1960s by a number of gurus, spiritual leaders and philosophers who promoted all things Indian. Their approach to life appealed hugely to many rock stars, like the Beatles and many celebrities as it contrasted starkly with the materialistic approach that predominated in the West at the time. For the West in general, however, yoga and meditation remained a mystery. Rather than being mainstream activities, they were taught by gurus who advocated strict discipline and a complete change in lifestyle; many teachers promoted vegetarianism -- which was quite radical a few deca des ago! Most people however, couldn't see the point in twisting the body into strange animal like configurations.

The West thus interpreted yoga as a series of exercises and thought of it in much the same way as other forms of physical activities and gymnastics. What's more, many people worried it would take years to master the many complicated positions. But the fact is that yoga is a suitable form of exercise and relaxation for everyone of all ages and abilities and it is safe.

Over the last few decades yogic exercise has become increasingly popular. Thanks to the efforts of some celebrities, together with the modern preoccupation with fitness and stress management. Yoga has become a household name and is now an established form of physical exercise. Yet, in its original form, yoga is so much more than just a system of exercise. For those in the know, yoga is a whole way of life, encompassing diet, massage, relaxation and meditation.

It regulates your breathing, it increases your energy, helping to overcome fatigue, it stretches and activates most of the muscles in the body, even some involuntary ones, removing the lactic acid that forms 'knots' within them. It relieves aches and pains in the joints and alleviates spinal problems. It improves your posture, and the circulation of blood and lymph and cleanses the body. It even exercises the mind as it calms and de-stresses you. As well as being a great way to stay in shape, it also promotes the body's natural healing powers, and can be used by anyone to treat a wide range of health problems, both physical and emotional – hence the description "therapeutic".

First it enhances breath control. Oxygen is essential to life. We can survive for a while without food or water, but not without air. We need oxygen to metabolise the food we eat and to create energy. On average, people breathe, 16 to 18 times a minute (although children may breathe slightly faster due to their higher metabolic activity). This is generally an involuntary process, meaning that most of the time you are not aware that you are doing it. Most of us breathe too shallowly and too fast, which can unfortunately result in major health problems.

There is a constant theme running through the philosophies of the major exercise routines of the world, typically yoga, Bates Method for the eyes, the Alexander Technique, Pilates, walking on uneven surfaces etc. They all build on the reconstitution of the control channels between brain and muscles in order to eliminate bad habits. In Hatha yoga, breathing is linked to physical movements so as to involve the subconscious brain. This alerts the brain to the ideal postures adopted and makes those patterns part of everyday habits.

Yogic (Hatha) Breathing

When you breathe normally, only about two thirds of the air in your lungs are expelled on exhalation and replaced when you inhale. The other third remains stagnant in your respiratory system because the lungs and the bronchial tract do not collapse totally during exhalation. When you practice yogic breathing, however, you can replace more of the air in your lungs. Yogic breathing is deeper and more efficient, and therefore more beneficial to the body.

Yoga teaches you to breathe slowly and deeply, helping you to deal with stress. The more anxious, you are, the more erratic your breathing. If you voluntarily slow your breathing into a deep rhythmic pattern, prolonging the time between inhalation and exhalation, oxygen absorption becomes more efficient. The blood returning to the heart from the lungs is therefore more enriched with oxygen, which triggers the brain to slow the heart rate. This can really help to calm you down by improving the oxygen supply to your brain. It helps to keep your brain cells healthy and active, which is particularly important as you grow older -- your brain tissues need three times more oxygen than the rest of your body. The two exercises, which I therefore recommend to start any yoga session, are Cleansing Breath and Alternate Nostril Breathing.

Cleansing Breath, (should not be attempted if you have high blood pressure, abdominal and hiatus hernia, and stomach ulcer, or prolapsed organs in the lower abdomen.

1. Stand or sit comfortably with your arms relaxed by your sides. Straighten your upper back and pull your shoulders back. Close your mouth and look straight ahead. Breathe in, fully through your nose.

2. Breathe out quickly, pulling your stomach in. Pause between breaths for a second or so and then repeat it again. Taking your time.
    Repeat 25 times. Relax for 10 minutes.

Alternate Nostril, Breathing

1. Sit cross-legged, if you can, on a straight-backed chair. Tap the index and middle fingers of your right hand into your palm. Place your thumb on your right nostril to close it and breathe in deeply through your left nostril.

2. Close your left nostril with your finger and release your thumb. Breathe out, completely through your right nostril. Feel your chest muscles relaxing and your shoulders dropping away from your neck as you exhale. Then breathe in through your right nostril.

3. Close your right nostril, release your finger and breathe out through the left nostril. You have now completed one cycle.

4. Continue for 3 to 5 minutes. Then relax for a few minutes.

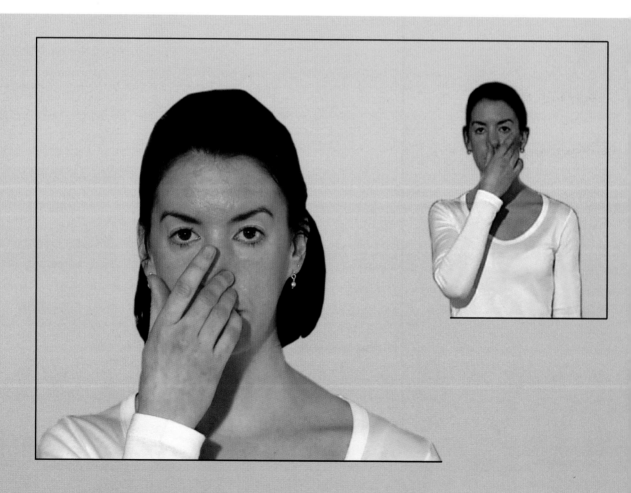

Yoga Involving the Neck

Many yoga exercises impinge upon the neck, while not being designed specifically for it.

Prone Exercises

LIE ON YOUR STOMACH

Cobra-full

1. Place your palms flat on the floor beside your shoulders.

2. Take a deep breath in, lift your torso up and look up to the ceiling. The entire body is arched back with the help of the back muscles and the arms give it minimal support.

3. Breathe out, and gently return to the original position with forehead on the floor.

Repeat this five times.

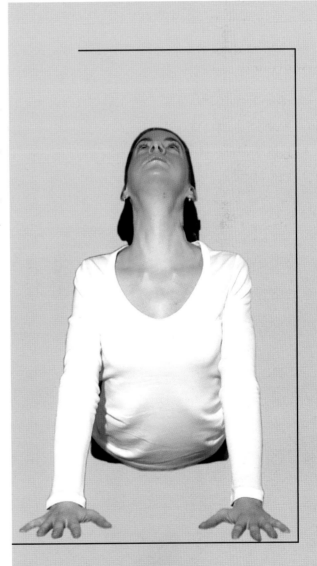

Cobra-half

1. Put your elbows by your sides. Take a deep breath in and raise your head, looking up. Hold your breath for five seconds, and slowly come down, breathing out. The forehead should touch the floor. Repeats this five times.

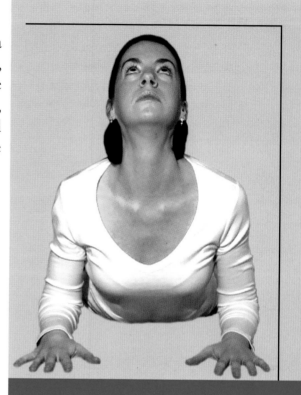

Self-traction

1. Put your hands together at the wrists and open your hands to make a bowl. Rest your chin on this bowl and place your palms on either side of your face. Your chin rests firmly on the base of the palms.

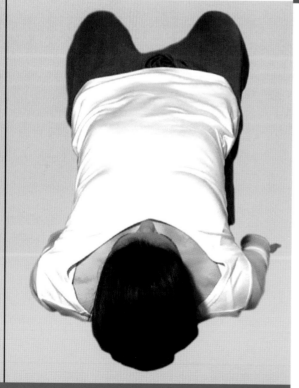

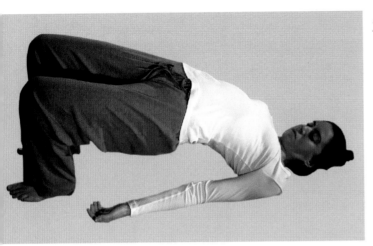

2. Join your elbows together, push them slightly forward and start to look up, so that you feel a traction of the neck. Breathe in and out very gently. On doing this a stretch should be felt in your entire spine. Hold this position for a couple of minutes.

Swing

1. Put both arms by your sides with palms under your thighs.

2. Take a deep breath in and raise your torso as well as your legs up in the air. Hold your breath in this position.

3. Arch your back, to look up and stretch your toes out. You should feel tightness along the back muscles, the seat muscles and the hamstrings and calves. Hold this position for a count of five.

4. Return to the normal position, breathing out again and placing your forehead on the floor.

Repeat five times.

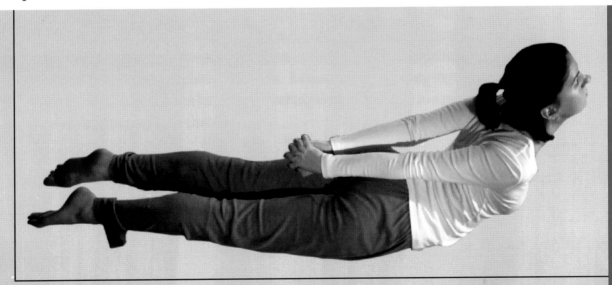

LIE ON YOUR BACK

Spinal Twist

1. Extend arms at shoulder level.

2. Bring knees up with feet on the floor.

3. Take a deep breath and turn your head to the left (ear should touch floor), while lowering your knees to the floor on the right (opposite direction).

4. Breathe out, and then breathe in and out very gently. As you do this you must make sure that your shoulders are flat on the floor. You should feel the twist in your spine and your knees will gradually descend to the floor as muscular tension is released from the lower back.

5. Repeat the exercise turning your head to the right and letting your knees come down to the floor on the left.

6. Repeat two or three times on each side.

This exercise will twist the spine to release spasm of muscles as well as help to align facet joints of vertebrae which get dislocated. This is a self-manipulative technique.

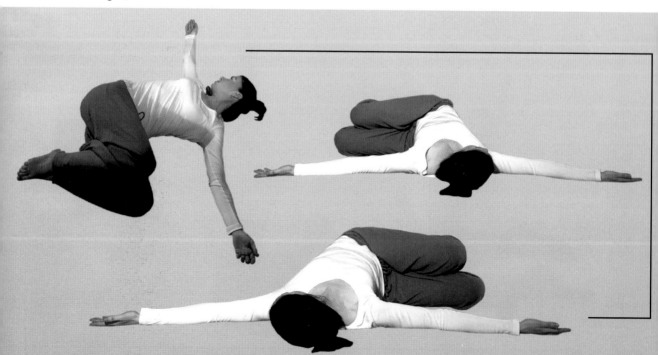

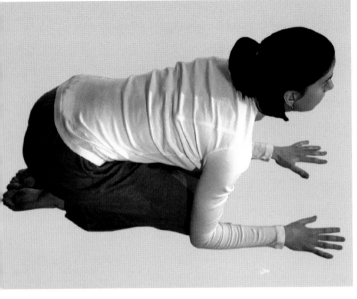

MIDWAY EXERCISES

Turtle-pose

1. Kneel and sit back on your heels. Place both elbows by the sides of the knees by bending forwards. Put your forehead on the floor.

2. Take a deep breath in and raise your head and look as far back as you can, keeping the elbows on the floor. Put your chest forwards. Hold your breath in this position for five seconds.

3. Slowly breathe out and return to the original position.

Repeat this five times.

STANDING EXERCISES

Arching back

1. Stand with feet together. Tighten your seat muscles. Breathe in.

2. Place both hands on the buttocks and push it forward. As you do this, look up, arching your back. Do not bend your knees while doing this.

3. Hold your breath for five seconds and return to the original position on breathing out.

4. Repeat this five times. You should be able to feel the tension in your lower back, and the release of it when you return to the original position.

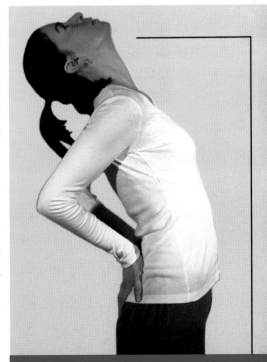

Arms arch

1. Stand with your feet together. Take a deep breath in and hold your breath.

2. Entwine your fingers behind your back, tighten your seat muscles and pull both arms down as if to touch your heels. Arch your back as you do this and look up. You should get the feeling that your back muscles and the muscles of your arms are taut.

3. Hold this position for a count of five. Breathe out and return to the normal position.

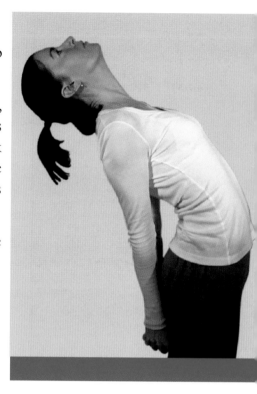

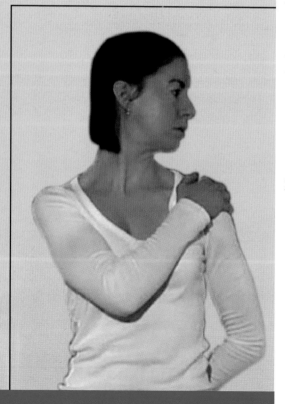

Yoga specifically for the Neck

Neck Twist

1. Look ahead and grip your right shoulder (in the middle, not at the extremity) with the left hand. Place the right arm behind your back.

2. Take a deep breath in and rotate your head towards the right, while simultaneously pulling the right shoulder forward with the left-hand. Hold your breath for five seconds. By doing this you will feel the stretch in the muscles of the right side of your neck and a release of tension in its joints.

3. Return to the original position.

4. Repeat the same with the other side.

5. Do this five times in each direction.

This exercise will strengthen the muscles of the neck, improve movement of the neck in both directions, releasing the stiffness and shifting vertebrae that are out of alignment back into their original positions. This often acts like self-manipulation.

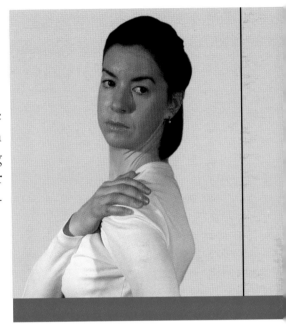

Head roll

1. Bend your head so that the chin touches your chest.

2. Rotate the head in a clockwise direction, making sure parts of your head (chin, lower jaw, back of the head) touch your chest and shoulder throughout its journey. This way, a total head roll is performed and the chances of dizziness are minimized.

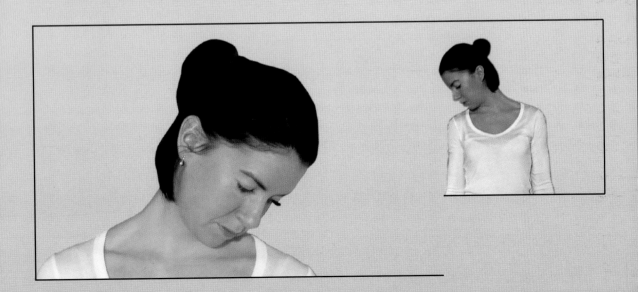

3.　Do this five times, and repeat in the anticlockwise direction.

This exercise will help to grind osteophytes or calcium deposits that so often settle on the joint services all around. This releases the joints from stiffness.

Whether it says so or not, breathing should be co-ordinated with each movement in all the exercises.

After your exercises, lie down and relax for five minutes.　Deep Relaxation is described fully in my Ultimate Back Book page 114, but basically it amounts to lying on your back in a quiet place with eyes closed; breathing deeply; concentrating on something abstract; being aware of your muscles becoming warm and relaxing all over your body; imagine your heart is slowing down. When ready take more deep breaths, open your eyes and rise slowly, avoiding anything stressful for as long as you can.

Therapeutic Yoga Today

I started this chapter with the beginnings of yoga 5000 years ago.　Relatively recently a new concept of yoga was created by an Indian guru, Jiten Kohi, and developed by an Indian doctor, Madan Kataria, who describes it in his book Laugh For No Reason.　It employs self triggered laughter, which is physical rather than humorous, and has become known as "Laughter Yoga".　The detail can be found on the Internet.　It can be performed by one person but is particularly effective in groups and has, for example, become widespread in homes for the elderly.　It can be regarded as an extension of yoga breathing bringing more oxygen to the body and the brain.　Obviously the oxygen has to reach the subconscious brain via the vertebral arteries, which have to be functioning properly if the exercise is to be fully effective.

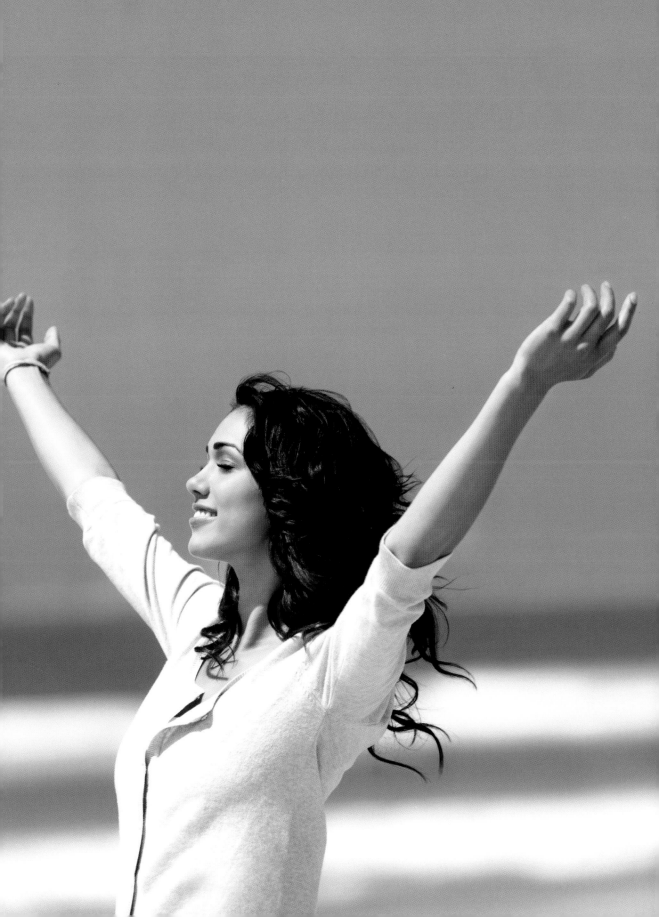

CHAPTER 17

Where to go for Treatment

The Ali Technique is one of the best tools for treating the neck and restoring all its functions. The neck holds the head, helps it turn in different directions, protects the most vital blood vessels and nerves, facilitates the nourishment and protection of the brain by regulating the circulation of cerebro spinal fluid and maintains the crucial link between the brain and the rest of the body. The neck is the most vital structure of the body and its functions have to be continually supported.

The Ali Technique is in practice, a family art of treatment. My brothers, some nephews and cousins, distant relatives, a few members of my village near Calcutta, some doctors who trained under me, some staff at The Castel Monastero Spa in Tuscany, and my sons know the technique. Previous staff therapists of my Integrated Medical Centres in London and New Delhi, and my Sagoor Charity Clinic in The Kangra Valley in the Himalayas follow my technique. My family members, however, know the finer aspects of my technique. I am proud that it is predominately a family art of healing. What pleases me most is that The Ali Technique will survive and continue to bring relief to the thousands we treat.

The massage technique described in the previous chapter, demonstrated in various DVDs and explained in my books is adequate for relief of many symptoms of the Ali Syndrome and maintenance of the functions of the neck. Read and watch the various aspects of the technique in my books, website and DVDs.

Here are other methods that help in the treatment of some of the symptoms of The Ali Syndrome and in preventing them:

1. Sports Massage. Qualified therapists who treat sports injury with massage.

2. Deep Tissue Massage.
3. Shiatsu of the neck and shoulder areas.
4. Osteopaths and Chiropractors who use massage first and manipulation later.
5. Thai Massage.
6. Ayurvedic, Head and Neck Massage.
7. Traction of the neck with low weights and controlled intermittent traction in extreme cases where massage therapy is not available.
8. Highly qualified Acupuncturists who are able to relieve neck tension.

All the above Practitioners and Therapists should be properly qualified and have minimum five years experience in a clinic or reputable Spa or Health Centres.

Please check my website for the list of Therapists who are directly or indirectly trained by me or my family members.

www.drmali.com

Shortly after the release of this book, Training courses will be offered to doctors, nurses, osteopaths, physiotherapists, qualified massage and sports injury Therapists.

Hopefully, there will be more therapists.

Here are the contact details of our centres:

Integrated Medical Centre
121, Crawford Street, London, W1U 6BE
info@integratedmed.co.uk

Integrated Medical Centre
D-40, East of Kailash, New Delhi-110065
Phones: +91-11-4652 2945
imc-delhi@msn.com

Castel Monastero
Near Siena, Tuscany, Italy
www.castelmonastero.com

For training courses contact:
info@theneckconnection.com

Other Neck Connections

The neck is located below the cranium, which houses the Headquarters of the nervous system - the computer centre. From the space below each of the seven cervical vertebrae a pair of nerves emerge from the spinal cord. The top three nerves "feed" or "innervate" the back of the head (occiput), the upper part of the neck and the area behind the ear. The next three, C3, C4 and C5 (cervical 3rd, 4th and 5th) innervate the lower portion of the neck and the shoulder. Finally, the vertebrae below these, C6 – C7 and the 1st and 2nd thoracic vertebrae supply nerves to the arms, hands and fingers.

Animals (our ancestors) walked on all fours so the thumb pointed up and the little finger pointed below. Hence, nerve root impingement at the cervical spine due to disc degeneration or calcium deposit around cervical joints can cause neurological symptoms going down to the fingers. Thus, if there is tingling, pain or numbness in the little finger then the nerve irritation is taking place at the level of C7 (7th cervical level). If it is the middle, ring and little fingers, altogether, then the roots at the level of C5 – C6 are scratched or irritated. If it's the index finger that is giving trouble, the C2 – C3 nerve root is involved. If it's the thumb then C6 is involved. Shoulder and deltoid pain, burning or numbness is due to the involvement of the C5 – C7 nerve roots. If the pain is in the back of the skull it's C2 – C3.

Thus compression of nerve roots emerging from the spinal cord at the neck level can cause pain, burning, tingling, electric currents and numbness in the occiput, neck, shoulder, arm and fingers. Usually if the nerve is severely pressed for a long time, and the nerves begin to lose their conductivity, the result is numbness (loss of feeling). The other symptoms are due to active irritation or compression. After a while, the damage to nerve roots is almost permanent, leading to 'wrist drop' which is due to loss of motor power.

The cervical vertebrae have disks to cushion them. These are located between the bodies of the vertebrae. If there is any whiplash, trauma or continuous wear and tear, these discs bulge and can scratch or irritate nerve roots, causing the above symptoms.

If one suffers from osteoporosis, the initial bone loss starts at the level of the neck, which is the most "stressed" part of the spine. This bone loss and the degeneration of the discs cause the neck to shrink. The person loses height. Later, bone loss may appear in the hip and lower spine. When the neck, shrinks, there is often a lot of nerve irritation at random. Women, who are more prone to suffer from osteoporosis, get all sorts of nerve pains, tingling, burning, numbness etc in the neck, shoulder, arms, hands and fingers. The vertebral arteries are also compressed and, as a result, the patient suffers from extreme fatigue, dizziness, imbalance, tinnitus and anxiety.

Sometimes the degenerated discs bulge into the spinal canal, rather than protrude out. This causes stenosis or narrowing of the spinal canal. Occasionally the bulge may touch or damage the spinal cord causing serious neurological problems.

A lady in her 70s came to see me with some strange sensations in her leg. She often lost power in her left foot while walking and tripped.   Sometimes she had to take extra care while climbing stairs as, for no apparent reason, her foot would drop and she would trip. I examined her and found no apparent cause of any back problem. I suspected that something was wrong with her neck. She had frequent headaches and dizziness. I sent her for an MRI of the neck. The result showed that a bony growth was touching and indenting the spinal cord at C6 – C7 level. I recommended she go for neurosurgery. This cured her problem.

Sylvester Stallone ,the very famous Hollywood star who is one of the top action heroes, took numerous direct hits on the face and head while filming of Rocky and Rambo films. He had sustained heavy injuries to the neck and shoulder areas. The pain was excruciating that he had to wear a neck brace to sleep at night. He was on the strongest painkillers you could find. Surgery was the only option. After some serious convincing from friends , he invited me to Los Angeles , I started working on his neck muscles , facet joints, tendons and ligaments twice a day. The pain was severe and I was lucky not to be punched by this strong man. After 6 days the pain was gone. He was greatly relieved.

Shah Rukh Khan , known as the King of Bollywood, is an incredible man of courage, tolerance and great intelligence. He went to the same chain of Christian Brother's School as I did. As an actor he did many of the stunts himself and therefore had to endure several injuries . In one film , for a more dramatic effect , he kicked the ground to scoop some dirt and throw it on the face of a wicked villain. Little did he know that there was a stone in the ground. He smashed his big toe and gave a perfect shot . He is a great dancer and years of repetitive injuries gave him some knee problems. He continues to do action scenes with a strained knee joint. Jumping from a tall building, moving between two trains running at full speed while being suspended from a crane, doing somersaults etc are not easy.

His neck injuries were top of the list. In one movie 'Dil Se' he danced on top of a moving train. While filming this song he had to move his neck sideways several thousands of times in a Sufi ritual, like those performed by Whirling Dervishes. In another film 'Devdas' the death scene was dramatic. He lay dead on the grass and his body was discovered in the early hours of the morning. To get the perfect morning light , the director shot this important scene for 11 days , filming only a few minutes a time. A fly was shown settling on his face as he lay motionless. This scene put a lot of strain on his neck muscles as he had tighten them and remain motionless.

In another movie , he ran across the airport check-in area to stop his wife from boarding a plane. They parted company the previous night. He jumped over a train of trolleys and landed on his back causing severe injury to the neck.

I was treating him for his neck and gave him much relief. The later injuries made the discs in the neck pinch the nerves. He had excruciating pain going down his left arm. Finally Mr. Crockard his Neuro-Surgeon , decided to operate . The pain continued so on the 2nd day after the surgery , Mr. Crockard gave me permission to treat him to alleviate the pain . He was in hospital then . I had never treated anyone so soon after surgery . Finally I got the pain under control. I treated him for a month while his nerve roots healed. He played monopoly with his friends while I treated him.

An Internationally known President of a famous luxury goods company was dining with the late Princess Diana and David Tang , a well-connected Hong Kong Entreprenuer. David has been a friend for 25 years or so. The gentleman complained of excruciating pain in his neck , shoulder and arm . He was going in for surgery . David, immediately called me. I was in the Palace of an Arab Head of State and had mistakenly forgot to switch off the phone. He ordered me to return to London "immediately" (David is always funny and very witty). I explained where I was.

I saw the gentleman after a few days . He was very sceptical as he had seen top specialists and they all suggested surgery .After the very first session he had some relief . He gave me the benefit of the doubt and invited me to his summer house.

I put him on a diet , treated him with my hands and gave him some exercises. The pain disappeared after a week and he came of all drugs as he would sleep comfortably. He became one of my greatest advocates. Through him I saw dozens of very important people all over the world. I am deeply indebted to him for appreciating my technique and skill. Sometimes you need angels like him to get you to where you are. So many people were saved from back and other operations because of him. Some was suffering from 'incurable' conditions.

Like all joints, the facet joints of the cervical spine are subject to arthritis. Most frequently it is due to wear and tear or old age. Sometimes, it is due to rheumatoid arthritis. The joints become very stiff and painful. Early morning stiffness of the neck is a predominant symptom. Blood tests can prove a positive rheumatoid factor. I use my JOINT OIL to ease these symptoms.

Sometimes the neck can go into spasm, on one side. You then get a "crooked neck". This condition is called Torticollis. It often happens due to sleeping awkwardly at night. You wake up in the morning with a crooked neck. I have also seen Torticollis in a few patients in India, due to drug reaction. There used to be a drug for nausea, which often caused Torticollis. You had to inject an antidote to cure the symptom. Neck massages and heat poultices are good treatments for Torticollis.

A well known Hollywood actor had a car accident in which he stretched the nerves of the neck. As a result there was paralysis in one arm. With excellent physiotherapy his one arm began to move but his hands remained out of actions. I met him at an event almost 3 years later and asked him if I could take a picture with him for my sons. He kindly agreed. Then I asked him casually, if he had any health problem. He told me about the accident, the excruciating pain he had in his arm and the loss of movement in his hand. I began to treat him in full glaze of hundreds of guests. As he is world famous, everyone saw what I was doing. After the first session he slept very well, without much pain. I saw him again for 2 hrs. the following day and explained what I did. He said "I trust you". I went to Los Angeles a few times and treated his neck and arm. The wrist and fingers began to move and the horrible pain disappeared.

Case Histories where Spontaneous healing with The Ali Technique took place

Improved blood supply to the subconscious brain improves general healing. Again, by using logic, we can see how that works. If the Pituitary-Hypothalamus region controls all autonomous functions in the body, then it must also control healing.

An English woman in her late forties came to me with a fracture in her tibia bone of the right leg. She had a compound fracture with many splinters. I don't remember how she did it. For three years, the fracture hadn't healed. She was on plaster for almost a year. She was desperate as she couldn't walk properly, had put on weight and there was pain. At first, I said I couldn't help her but she insisted I use some of my "magic" and used my healing hands. I said I would try. I changed her diet, asked her to drink marrow bone soup (marrow bone boiled in slow heat for 2 hours to get the calcium and gelatine out), eat fresh fruits and green salad. I gave her weekly treatment of the neck and back and also massage the thigh and calf muscles (avoiding the fractured area). After 8 weeks she went to have an x-ray. The doctors were very pleased in the hospital as they saw evidence of new bone tissue. After 8 more weeks the bone healed. It was amazing but it worked.

When Wayne Rooney, the English football star, who plays for Manchester United Team, had a fracture of the metatarsal bone in his foot, the whole nation was in despair. It was just before the 2006 World Cup and he was one of the main goal scorers. I suggested my treatment through a Press release, covered only by The Sun newspaper. Then I was called on Sky News TV to give my suggestion. They interviewed me for 5 minutes to explain what I could do tom make him heal quickly. Hundreds of patients with fractures of various types contacted me after the TV interview. I gave my treatment plan: Neck massage, Diet and gentle exercise.

An Indian lady could not get a Canadian Visa to join her husband. She failed the crucial medical test because she had an infected left Humerus bone (arm). The infection

(Osteomalacia) produced pus that oozed out from the arm. She used to dress the wound and was on antibiotic permanently. Her husband had a job in Toronto and wanted to settle down there. The wife came to see me in desperation from Punjab, some 8 hours journey from Delhi. I didn't promise her anything and suggested a diet of juices, cottage cheese, soaked almonds and some protein powder. She was a strict vegetarian and so I had to suggest cottage cheese as the main source of protein and calcium. I taught her relative how to do neck massage.

After 6 months she came to visit me in my Delhi clinic. She showed me a piece of bone in a jar, she also gave me some x-rays of her arm which showed the process of healing in sequence. Her body rejected the piece of infected bone and you can see it in progress. I was surprised as I recommended a "fluke" treatment. I still have those magical x-rays which I have used in my public lectures. Her sores healed and she now lives in Canada.

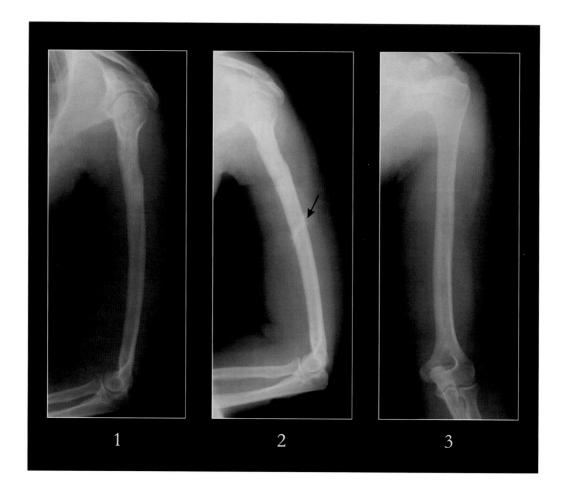

1   2   3

A cloth merchant from Delhi requested me to see his ailing father who had brain tumour (Glioma). I was reluctant to treat him but he begged me to visit him so that his father will feel confident. I flew to Amritsar in Northern India from Delhi and went to see the patient. When I saw him, he was having one of the frequent seizures. His face was swollen and he lost a lot of weight as he had constant nausea and headaches. It was obvious he was dying and there was nothing I could do. Since I had gone there, I thought I should at least try to make him feel better.

I suggested, Khichdi rice (rice cooked with lentils, till it becomes like porridge, kedgree rice), carrot and apple juices and yoghurt. He was vegetarian so I couldn't even suggest eggs as a source of protein. I demonstrated the neck and shoulder massage to a relative. I suggested they did the massage three times a day. I also suggested some liquid multi-vitamins with minerals. I suggested, he ate one mouthful at a time over a hour.

After just 2 weeks, the son came to see me in my clinic. He had visited his father over the weekend and he responded positively to the treatment. His seizures stopped and he could eat normal food without being sick. I felt good. When you are young and have less experience, every success story makes you feel elated.

A few months later, he was brought to Delhi to see me. I compared his CT scan with the first one and there was a definite reduction in the tumour size.

A few months later, he came to see me again. He was perfectly normal. I took him to Aggarwal x-ray and scan centre in central Delhi. After the CT scan, Dr Aggarwal who knew me well asked me what I did. He was surprised, as the Tumour had completely disappeared. He said he had never seen anything like that in his entire career.

I didn't use any medicine so the general treatment with neck massage triggered self-healing. I still have the CT scans and I have used them in my lectures.

A little boy of 1 & ½ years with Down Syndrome was brought to see me by her mother. She said she would try anything, I suggested to help the child. Every week he came for his neck and back therapy. After 6 months, he started to speak a few words. He became very alert, his focus was good, he developed noticeable communication skills, hardly suffered colds and cough and is a very cheerful boy.

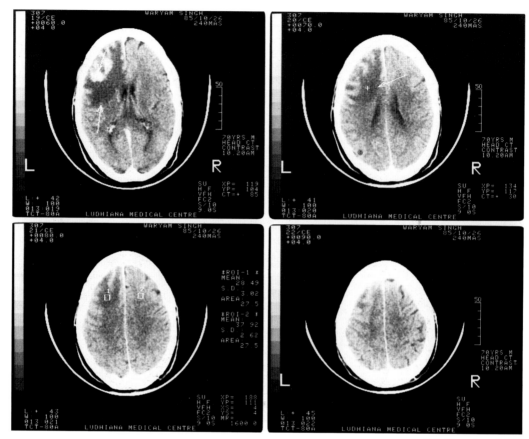

26 October 1985

Its his 3rd year of treatment and he has almost caught up with his milestones developed. He has a genetic problem linked to a chromosome defect and yet he had noticeable improvement in his physical and emotional state. He didn't have any birth injury or neck trauma. There is no neck connection here.

Several cases of Multiple Sclerosis are under our treatment. The neck treatment has helped them to go into remission. Sometimes, there is no limit to any birth injuries or head and neck trauma.

One young lady with confirmed MS is under our treatment using The Ali technique. She is now lives in India where it is quite hot in the summer, something that aggravates the symptoms of muscle weakness, coordination fatigue etc. She gets occasional tingling or pain in the legs due to normal backache or sciatica, but with treatment that gets quickly resolved. Its almost 10 years now and she has

21 April 1986

come off steroids and is in long term remission. She hasn't had a scan to see if the plaques or "white spots" are still there in the brain.

After 10 years ago, when I used to write a column for The Mail on Sunday's coloured supplement the YOU magazine, a patient asked me for advice on Cancer therapy. In the column I wrote about diet, juices, neck massage, meditation and some supplements as adjuvant therapy to normal medical treatment with Radio and Chemotherapy.

After a few weeks as official from The Westminster Council's Health Department in London came to see me. He served me a letter to say that I broke the 1930 Law on promoting Cancer Therapy, which was not officially accepted. I was expecting a heavy fine. I said that because I moved into the UK in 1991 to live here, I was not aware of any law that restricts me to publicly express my views on a health matter. I also argued that I did not recommend any chemicals or herbs for cancer and nor I did I claim to have a cure for cancer. For chronic disease like Cancer, Rheumatoid Arthritis, Multiple Sclerosis etc. if I notice a notable improvement in a patient's condition, I say that disease has gone into remission. Its not a cure even though I feel that I might have cured it.

As a well know practitioner of Integrated Medicine, a lot of Cancer patients come to me for advice. I tell them to go through the normal medical plan of therapy with surgery when possible, chemotherapy and radiotherapy as all three have a great role to play in controlling the cancer. I suggest a therapy to counteract the side effects of such drugs and focus of well-being and feel-good factor. My belief is that if we counteract the effect of chemo or radio therapy, the chances are that the body will be able to spring back to health. A strict diet (organic food where possible), vegetable and fruit juices for additional vitamins, minerals and enzymes, massage of the whole body particularly the neck and shoulder areas, meditation or relaxation, some supplements and herbal remedies (for candida, energy, digestive disturbances, liver functions etc) helps the body and the mind. The neck massage improves sleep, eliminates symptoms like nausea, fatigue, headaches, insomnia etc (after chemotherapy) and gives a boost to the energy. This way the patients can tolerate these strong therapies better. My programme continues even after these therapies for 5 years or so. Then we can see true remission.

A lady with breast cancer was given 2-3 months to live as the chemotherapy didn't work at first and the side effects were horrendous (sickness, fainting, anxiety). Its her 4th year now and she goes through regular check-up without any sign of cancer anywhere.

I must warn, that my treatment only helps patients to cope with the conventional therapies, which must destroy the cancer cells. Later, my therapy helps with comfortable recuperation. That is what helps patients to go into remission.

A lady with Caposi Sarcoma with positive HIV had the surgery. The tumour in the face (Caused by Herpes Virus, complication of AIDS) was removed. She was infected by a boy friend. I suggested a trial therapy of diet, neck massage and supplements. She had that regularly for 6 months. Actually, she went on to study Ayurvedic Medicine to understand her condition better. It's almost 10 years and she has not active lexicons in the body. She is HIV positive but in remission.

A woman in her early fifties had a lot of stress in her life. A divorce, loss of a powerful job , financial problems, loneliness etc, ruined her life. She had total Alopecia and lost all her hair and eyebrows. She wore a head scarf and pencilled her eyebrows. This caused more stress as she stopped socialising and lost all hopes of getting a job. She was severely depressed .She saw several specialists and took steroids but nothing helped.

Months went by and she finally decided to take her own life. She went on a small mainline station where high speed trains passed. When she arrived she learnt that the long distance trains were cancelled. She returned home and cried for hours.

In the days that followed , someone spoke to her about me. She came to see me. I was really touched by her story . I gave her a lot of courage and told her to change her diet , have regular neck treatments and do yoga. She was so impressed that she followed my instructions very carefully. After a few weeks , the hair started to appear on her scalp. This encouraged her to follow the programme religiously.

She went on my Himalayan trip and stayed on for a few more weeks .She was Indian but lived abroad all her life. With great enthusiasm she studied the culture, local tradition and their lives.

After almost a year , her eyebrows and hair came back totally. She had made a decision that at her daughter's wedding she would not use a scarf or a wig. So she did. Today she is the proud grandmother of a beautiful girl.

Whenever her grand daughter has any problems like , cradle cap that doesn't heal , colic , constipation ,flu, etc , she comes to see me. She was born with with forceps and has had some problems . Little Mariam has daily neck and body massage and is growing up to be a delightful and healthy child .I am very fond of her.

These are individual cases but even one case is symbolic. It goes to prove that the treatment has some very positive effect on the body. I will continue to accept difficult cases where medicine fails because deep in my heart I believe that I have discovered a Panacea of health. Any help I can offer to such chronic patients who are in agony is a bonus. I am doing my job as a doctor, the best I can. All I believe in is Hippocratic preaching "Physicians do no harm". My treatment has not harmed anybody, even if it has not helped some. It is a natural treatment after all using massage, and exercises.

My Own Experience

So why did I write this book? I have had the compelling desire to reveal the importance of truly understanding and caring for the neck since I was a young student in Boarding school. I was studying hard and suffering severe insomnia, hyperactivity and headaches. It was a Christian Brother who became concerned for my welfare and showed me the way. Now I want to pass on

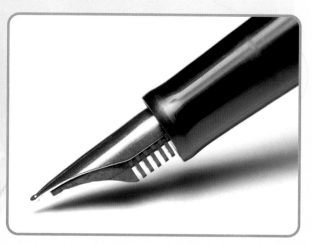

what I have learned through my own experiences of neck injuries - hence this book.

It all started with my maternal grandfather, who was both a doctor and a homeopath. He was a great believer in natural birth and non-invasive methods of treatment. In fact he was a true integrated medical doctor. He preferred to use homeopathic remedies rather than allopathic medicines.

I was the first born in the family and my grandfather insisted that my mother had the best midwife in the area. I was delivered in the family home near Calcutta. My mother told me the labour was long and difficult. I realized later that my head must have been stuck in the birth canal. The contractions must have squashed my neck periodically over several hours. That is not an uncommon occurrence.

In theory I should have had some birth injuries to the neck which would have led to a weak immune system, eczema, lack of concentration etc. However my grandfather did what was the tradition in India. For forty days both my mother and I received care from the midwives, who are called 'Dais' in India.

In the holy City of Banares on the Ganges, said to be the oldest city in the world, there was a school that trained these Dais. They were taught to care for both the mother and the new born. They made sure every thing was hygienic and the new born was fed on time, bathed, sunbathed, dressed and handled while transferring to the mother. The mother was also taught child care and allowed the necessary time to recuperate fully. She learned how to prepare a good diet and to take enough rest to produce the best quality milk for the newborn.

The massage of the neck and the caution in handling the head and neck, rectified all the trauma and damage the newborn may have endured at birth. At the end of the 40 day period, the baby was able to hold the head up with more strength. Massage plays an important role in restoring good blood flow to the fast developing brain. The result is that the child feels well, does not suffer from colds or coughs, develops at the right rate and is generally happy and alert.

My mother told me I was brought up according to my grandfather's instructions, breastfed and given the daily massage the Dai taught almost every day for the first year. She said I never suffered from colic, diarrhea, infection, rash, bloating or any of the trials that new babies are so often heir to. I crawled and walked early and was a quick learner.

Could it be that my memory developed well because of that massage of the neck and shoulder area? For example, on my first birthday my grandfather gave me a present, I later learned was a gold chain and gold waistband with semiprecious stones on it. There were a large number of family and friends gathered in his mansion to celebrate the birthday occasion. I remember being aware of my mother's deep distress when one of the guests stole the precious gift. I was conscious too of my grandfather's fury. It left a clear impression on me. The theft was never solved and it was a very unpleasant incident as many guests left without attending the family feast.

I can remember another incident too that happened when I was about eighteen months old. I was sitting in a truck surrounded by many people shouting "Vote for Ali". My father, a politician, in those days stood for Bengal elections and I was taken by someone for the campaign trip. My father won the election and we had many visitors to the house. One was Dr. B.C.Roy, the first chief minister of

Bengal who later became my ideal. He used to diagnose patients by looking at tell-tale signs of the body, tongue, pulse and eyes. Today part of my own diagnosis follows this technique. Dr Roy received his MRCP in London because he diagnosed small pox in an immigrant patient at its early stage when no other professor could.

I was a good student and came first in my class at school. The son of a wealthy businessman died of leukaemia in my school. The father was very disheartened. He set up a scholarship in his honour for the student who achieved the best percentage of marks. I was the first recipient of that scholarship. I often attribute the fact that I was able to reach outstanding achievements of scholarship to the fact that I had such good care at my birth. It was the basis of my success in life.

When I look at early photographs of myself, I observe that my left eye was smaller than the right. That is an indication that I sustained some significant birth injuries and yet I didn't have any of the complications that I have mentioned in this book. The early treatment was my saviour and damage to the nerve (the 7th cranial nerve, a facial nerve) was as near completely rectified. Sometimes when I am tired, I do find my left eye slightly shut and the asymmetry of the eyes is noticeable.

When I was eight years old I was sent to boarding school. The school building had been a Military Hospital during the First World War. It was there that they used to treat the British soldiers who were wounded on the Eastern front. The school was run by Christian Brothers who were strict but very caring. I was there for eight years and during that time had suffered two distinct injuries. Once when I was playing grass hockey, the ball hit me hard on the nose and it bled profusely. I was dizzy afterwards for several days. I enjoyed outdoor sports and activities. It was when I was in class 10 that I decided that I wanted to box. I realized I must prepare myself. I joined a group who used to go for a jog at 5.30 am every day, followed by exercises. For breakfast we had a meal of soaked horse gram (pulses) ,a rich source of protein used by wrestlers and sportsmen in Asia. I also took raw egg for stamina. I was tall, skinny and had long arms for my weight; I thought I had all the advantages for a boxer. The very first time I was in the ring I was punched by my opponent on the nose; I had flashes before my eyes, and almost lost balance. My neck arteries were shaken – and the fight was stopped. I could not smell very well for days and the olfactory system must have received a real jolt. If the trauma was in the nerve ending of the nose I would have had total loss of smell but when it was receiving a strong smell, the trauma affected the olfactory (smell) centres in the brain. That was typical of the Neck Connection.

I was still young and very active so the symptoms disappeared quite quickly. It was a year later I started getting insomnia. I would wake up at 3 am sharp and would not be able to sleep until 5 am or so. This happened on most nights. Initially I would try to divert my mind, I counted sheep, imagined that I was flying like a bird over valleys and fields, sometimes these helped but generally the routine remained the same.

Being a conscientious student I would go down at night to the study hall to study. The schoolmasters were confident I would achieve a rank in the final school leaving board examination conducted by the University of Cambridge. Our principal, Brother Whiting, a very caring missionary from Adelaide, patrolled every night to be sure that all was well in the dormitories. He became aware that I didn't sleep well. He frequently came down to the study room and encouraged me to go to bed to get some sleep. He knew that I was determined to do well in my studies and thought I was overly industrious. He did not realize that I was suffering from serious insomnia.

Just before my board examination was due to begin I could not sleep at all. The tension of the examination exacerbated the situation. One night when Brother Whiting was doing his rounds I confessed my situation to him. He realized then that I was suffering from sleep deprivation and immediately spoke to the school nurse who gave me some bitter potion to drink at bed-time. That gave me at least 3-4 hours sleep and then I would be wide awake again. It was almost two weeks before the exams and I still couldn't sleep well. Bro Whiting became very concerned that I was hyperactive and worried that I might fail my examinations.

My first exam was physics, which I answered well and scored 91 %. At around ten pm Brother Whiting came to my bed and gave me a neck and back massage. I'll never forget that moment. He was firm and so caring and I slept right through till the morning. From then on, before every examination, he would do the same for 5 to 10 minutes. It broke the cycle and gave me a vocation for life.

After the examination I went to Calcutta for a holiday to see my Mother. Nearly every night she gave me a massage of the neck and head. It had a wonderful effect and worked like magic, I was able to sleep again. Nowadays I work hard during the day with no time for reading or writing so I write books and articles at night. I have got into the habit of sleeping for only 4-5 hours. After a long flight I ask one of my brother therapists in the clinic to give me a neck massage, I never feel jet-lagged.

Over the years I have developed a system of treatment for my patients which has proved immensely successful. For more than 20 years I have been taking groups to the Himalayas for therapy. The effect of altitude, massage. yoga, walking and careful diet has a tremendous impact on healing.

We usually stay in Taragarh Palace Hotel in the Kangra Valley in India. About 10 years ago, the Prince of Kashmir, who owned the Palace, was rebuilding a house nearby that had remained unused for 60 years. Everyone had kept away as there were many stories about it being `haunted'. They believed the previous owner, whose spirit was evil, still influenced the premises. I wanted to see the house. The Prince's manager offered to take me there. On the first floor one could walk on to a terrace that gave a fabulous panoramic view of the mountains. I walked briskly to the terrace, I was anxious to see the view. As I did so my forehead hit the beam of the door and I stumbled and fell to the floor. I saw stars and felt very dizzy, rather sick and when I tried to focus, my vision was blurred. The manager who was showing me the house was extremely worried. I lay on the floor for a few minutes and then, aware of his concern, forced myself to get up slowly. I assured him that I was alright and not to worry although the dizziness continued and I had to lean against the wall. I was very perplexed. How could I hit that beam? It was a normal door, the beam was above my head, so what happened? I was told later that there had been a mysterious fire that severely burnt the house and ever since it had remained empty. The French mistress of the ruler of Bahawalpur, near Lahore in Pakistan, lived in that house before India's partition. I lay in bed for the rest of that day and slept deeply until I was woken up for dinner, where the others in the group told me I should have been more careful in a haunted house. By then my massage therapist had heard what had happened. I had some neck pain and soreness in the forehead I asked one of my therapists to massage my neck and I put a hot salt fomentation on it after which I slept very deeply. Next morning I woke up feeling better. There was no dizziness but a mild headache remained. Feeling somewhat weak I went downstairs for breakfast and later took a walk with the group and had some neck treatment in the evening. The dizziness gradually disappeared. The flight back home to London was comfortable but I had an unusual fatigue afterwards. Even though I traveled in Business Class, the jet lag was worse that time. Then I heard a continuous ringing in my right ear. It was tinnitus, another symptom of the Neck Connection. I immediately began to treat my neck myself, the tinnitus went after a few days of treatment. I did yoga regularly and focused on the neck exercises.

We never know when we will turn a corner and an event will take place that will affect our lives. Such an event happened to me one day on one of the walks on my Himalayas trips. As we took one path we were surprised to see it led to a collection of caves and beautiful waterfalls. We walked through to get to the complex. In the background behind us we could see the mighty snow-capped Himalayas and members of our party stopped frequently to take photos of the green fields with the mountains in the back-ground. It was one of the most spectacular, interesting and impressive walks I had ever been on. We were fascinated to discover that in one of the caves there lived a Holy man. He was in his eighties, wore simple clothes and had very long hair (about 1.5 metres). Here in the cave Baba Sant Ram meditated and lived his life. He had left the British army when he was 20 years old and had moved into the complex of interconnecting caves. It was here that for thousands of years other Holy men had lived. The paintings on the wall were evidence of past habitation. The Baba sage was highly gifted. He gave discourse on life, religion and spirituality. My visiting guests were amazed and enraptured. He asked one guest to press his left index finger with her hands. Baba then closed his eyes and told her quite accurately about her past, her circumstances and incidents that only she knew. The visitors were stunned by the visit and it was to become a regular part of my trips with patients to the Himalayas.

My Indian treks became an important part of my healing service. I decided to make a documentary film. I traveled around India interviewing various masters accompanied by a movie cameraman called Kedar. I interviewed the 90 year old world famous yoga master Iyengar and the 95 year old head of the Ramakrishna mission in Belur on the bank of the Hooghly River in Calcutta. I met so many exceptional men connected with health and spirituality. During our travels we went to the Kangra valley intent on filming Baba Sant Ram. We arrived at the Palace in the evening and I called the gatekeeper who knew him to take us to the caves to meet the Holy Man. I had felt deeply compelled to go and visit Baba. It was a huge shock therefore when they told me that he had died that very morning. I had felt compelled to go there - why now when it was too late? I was numbed.

The next morning I went to the caves to pay my last respects. Waiting there was his eldest son, Hari Singh. He expected me. He told me that his father had a premonition that I was coming, he had said that the doctor from London would be coming but that he would be too late. He had told his son about the bamboo bridge across the river for the villagers I had helped him build so that the villagers were able to cross, especially when the water level was high. That day, on that spot, I decided to open a charity clinic for the poor people in the area. I made the announcement to the family and to hundreds of villagers that had gathered for a prayer meeting for the Baba. We walked to the waterfall, a truly peaceful place, I still call it my paradise. As I walked down I fell sliding down the rocks. I felt a little unsteady. Was it an accident or a test of my intention?

A few days later, when my group arrived we went to the caves. My son Azeem was with me and as I walked from the waterfall towards the huge boulders where everyone was having their picnic lunch something strange happened. I tripped on a small crack on the floor of the huge cave and went flying in the air. I fell on my back into the pool full of rocks. I distinctly remember hitting the rock submerged in the pool and instantaneously jerking my head forward in a reflex. That saved my head from hitting the rock. Everybody rushed towards me to pull me out of the fall. What a lucky thing that was. I could have definitely had a serious injury then. The editor of this book was there with his wife Aileen. They saw the bizarre fall I had in the waterfall. It was as if I was flying over a high jump bar.

What saved me was that jerking reflex that pulled my head up. Sylvester Stallone once told me that when you are knocked down in a boxing match and land on your back the most dangerous injury is sustained by the neck. Before the back of your head hits the floor it swings forward in a reflex, injuring neck muscles. It is worse than whiplash which is a horizontal movement. The neck muscles in the front pull your heavy head up against the force of gravity so the strain is tremendous.

I was shocked and had a sinking feeling. I lay on a boulder. Everybody who was there including Azeem, was shocked too. We all thought of the worst scenarios of a spinal injury. I wondered if I had had a warning. Was this a message, a test or a warning about something? Certainly the inhabitants of that unique and isolated area had no medical support. What if they were taken ill, a child, a young woman or the elderly? What could I do to help? That evening I had a rare headache and felt very tired. I slept on a very thin pillow and fortunately my therapists knew what to do to the neck to prevent complications.

A month later, I was going to a friend's house for dinner and had a perfect example of the old saying `more haste, less speed'. I was already running late because of the heavy traffic but my car needed filling so I stopped at a petrol station on the way. Quickly I filled the tank and hurried towards the kiosk to pay. As I did so I rushed into a full length glass door, crash – a quite common accident these days. I hit my nose badly, it bled profusely and I was shocked and dizzy. The assistant at the till was very concerned and hurried over with tissues. After I paid the bill I went back and sat in my car for several minutes with my door open – I was dazed and my neck hurt. I pulled myself together and drove slowly to my friend's home and there put some ice cubes on the nose to stop the blood.

The truth is, apart from hurrying because I was late, my mind was elsewhere. My thoughts were far away in India. I was thinking about the caves and the Baba and my proposed clinic. That very morning I had passed the last barrier. I had committed myself to opening a clinic there. The agreement to buy the plot near the caves was signed. My life would never be quite the same again. It had been a very special day that ended in a big neck injury. Since that day much of my heart is there underneath the magnificent Himalayas in my clinic close to the caves which has grown from nothing to bring relief to the thousands of people who cannot afford good medical treatment. Everything is provided free for the people of the valley.

After these three injures in a row, I became more aware of the consequences and the health risks through injuries to the neck. I began to have treatment for the neck from time to time. I now understand that I too have a neck issue and I am convinced that if I didn't take care of it I would be in trouble. I do get tinnitus when I am tired, suffer from short term memory loss when I work non-stop for a few weeks in a row and have had blurred vision on occasion. Through good care that is all I suffer.

As a tall man I have hit my head on car doors, headboards of beds, low ceilings etc. and fortunately know what to do to come to my own rescue.

I have used the neck treatment to help myself, my family and thousands of patients. The results have been amazing. My sons Shahzad and Azeem know that whenever they get a cold or cough I use the neck massage to fix their weakened immune system. I use sinus oil, vitamins and minerals and give them breathing exercises. It always works for them. No antibiotics.

Recently Shahzad went to Peru and up to Machu Pichchu and Lake Titicaca at almost 4000 metres with some friends. I told him to use the neck massage technique. He always suffered from altitude sickness above 2000 metres . This time, thanks to the massage treatment, he had no problem at all. His friends didn't have any symptoms of altitude sickness, even though even though they were prone to it.

I spend a great deal of time traveling these days. Every week I fly from my Clinic in London to Florence to treat patients in the Castel Monastero Spa, a lovely resort in Tuscany. I fly to India, of course, and to many other countries. Along with long working hours all this has caused my neck to stiffen. Added to this I have had several severe knocks to my head and have also had neck injuries. I also had a typical whiplash injury as many drivers and passengers will have suffered from traffic accidents. A severe one happened to me when I stopped at the traffic lights on Park Lane in London.   A large white van hit me from the back at full force. I was jerked forward and injured my neck. It gave me a lot of pain, palpitations, fatigue and anxiety. All these affect my neck during my frequent flights. I suffer myself from the Ali Syndrome but my regular neck treatment and exercise keep everything under control. I am rarely ill with colds & flu so the immune system is strong and I have good energy.

My personal experiences of neck problems have gone a long way to convince me that my discovery, hypothesis and treatment are successful and unique. I have come to understand the matter thoroughly and can now openly discuss it with confidence and conviction.

In conclusion I cannot make my point about the importance of the neck more strongly than by telling you a story that touched me most deeply. It happened to one of my old pupil. Dasgupta did very well and was promoted to a high post in the Calcutta Port Trust. He lived with his wife and son in a beautiful apartment. Life was perfect. One day his son, while washing his face in the basin, raised his head and hit the tap. He immediately collapsed and lay unconscious on the floor. His mother rushed him to the hospital. He was dead on arrival. The tap had hit the back of the child's head, jolted the tender neck and the vertebral arteries developed a kink. The acute decrease in blood flow switched off the vital centers in the brain stem that control breathing and heart beat. The small boy's heart could beat no more.

Dasgupta sold his flat and went to live with his wife in a remote village near Darjeeling. He gave up his prosperous life and career and now dedicates himself to teaching underprivileged tribal children. He could no longer bear Calcutta, he felt peace and prosperity were not for him in this life. I felt compelled to write this book and that story completes the circle. I started by reminding my readers that a sharp blow to the neck can be fatal. By telling what happened to a personal friend I end with an example of that truth.

EPILOGUE

Yes, I have discovered the role of the vertebral arteries in the neck, in health and disease. An Italian surgeon, managed to cure several cases of Multiple Sclerosis by operating on the veins of the neck. There has been a lot of press about this. Following that some MS patients held pickets in Canada outside the offices of Medical Authorities there, demanding that more research should be done so that such treatment is available there. A professor in Leeds University in the UK, carried out some trials and proved that neck massages helped to lower High Blood Pressure. His explanation is that some "trigger points" in the neck had this amazing effect. I know why these results are puzzling scientist. There is a talk in Italy about carrying out Research on the neck arteries to see what else they can cure. I am glad that they are sniffing around for some clue.

I have an edge over all these scientists in treatment of numerous diseases with my technique . I started over 22 years ago and have tremendous experience on the role of these arteries. I have an additional advantage in that, I know what to do about it.

Currently, I am the Head of The Clinical Spa called Castel Monastero near Siena in Tuscany, Italy. It is a 1100 year old Monastery converted into a beautiful 75 rooms hotel with my Clinical Spa. I run my unique Health Programmes there. People come with a variety of health problems but the treatments are almost identical. They follow my diet, have my neck massage, additional fully body Marma massage (using points in the body), do yoga, drink my teas and walk or exercise. Sometimes specific remedies and supplements are used. The basic plan of treatment is the same and yet people get cured of fatigue, headaches, backaches, digestive problems, allergies, stress, weight gain, etc. They feel and look good. This proves that my Treatment Plan at the Spa has a cure-all effect. This integrated approach, combined with the Neck Treatment is my model of treatment.

Within 6 months the Spa has built a huge reputation. It is fully booked most of the time. The word is spreading very fast. This is direct proof that the treatment works. I know very well that I have written a controversial book and do expect a lot of challenges to my hypothesis. I am mentally ready for it. I have intentionally dropped names of famous people in many cases. These people will no doubt stand by me and give testimonials to prove that what I did was correct and that they benefited from my treatments.

I would like to see Research being carried out in future to prove that reduced blood flow to the brain can cause a variety of symptoms. So far, PET SCAN is the closest we got to detect the reduced radioactive glucose uptake by brain tissue. This injected glucose is carried by blood to various parts of the brain so its low density means low blood flow. In Chronic Fatigue Syndrome, PET scan proved general reduction of blood flow to the brain. Specific symptoms like Tinnitus, Blurred Vision, Nausea, Vertigo etc. will need more sophisticated scans to prove that. Thus we do not have the technology to prove that minute reduction of blood flow in smaller capillaries in the brain can cause symptoms of illness Moreover, the tests have to be carried out when the actual symptoms occur. Thus dynamic changes should be precisely recorded. If a person is dizzy, then one should record the changes in blood flow in the cerebellum as it happens. Some symptoms like Tinnitus blurred vision, fatigue etc. are continuous. The reduced blood flow may have led to these symptoms which didn't disappear when blood flow was somewhat restored. Headache would be a good symptom to study. It stays for a while but if blood circulation is restored (measurable) that symptoms would disappear.

When Galen (Greek-Roman Surgeon/Physician) discovered these arteries

2000 years ago, he didn't know what they did. He named them as Vertebral Arteries as they were found inside the cervical vertebral canals. He performed vivi section in live slaves. By cutting nerves, he knew their functions (vision, taste, hearing, smell) but cutting arteries would have had fatal consequences.

I faced the humiliation of being called a masseur for extensively using my hands to treat. As I had my main degree from the former Soviet Union, people often didn't recognise me as a doctor. All Medical Insurance Companies except Bupa International, refused to accept me as a provider or specialist of Complimentary Medicine and yet I saved them hundreds of thousands of pounds every year in expensive medical treatments. Patients often argued with them to claim the money back after getting cured of their chronic illnesses. Now I face the prospect of being challenged by these companies due to increase in claims by patients and under pressure from the medical establishment for bringing out a ridiculous idea that numerous diseases can be cured by treating the neck .I had to tell my story for the sake of the millions who are suffering due to accidents, traumas, excessive computer use, stress etc.

Like Gallen, these vertebral arteries will have to be studied in vivo (in live humans), which is highly unethical. My logical explanation therefore remains the only way to prove that there is a Neck Connection in many diseases.

Acknowledgements

The Neck Connection is a result of over 20 years of my work. I have been longing to share the astounding facts revealed here. I first wrote it, some 15 years ago. My dear friend and the Editor of several of my books, Ken Bridgewater, and his broadcaster wife Aileen, who live in Hong Kong, wanted me to publish then. However I waited because I was a novice in the world of writing. Today, I am now well known in the UK and Europe and am confident that I have gathered enough case histories and experience to prove my point. I tested my case in lectures for esteemed groups like WPO (World Presidents Organisation), on TV, in the weekly column of The Mail on Sunday and in discussions with discerning, learned people. I have taught groups of doctors who were converted into this doctrine.

I am grateful to those who believed in me, my friends, patients, students, readers, my sincere thanks to you. Without your feedback this book would not have been possible. I want to thank Ken Bridgewater for editing this book . I thank Yves Gougoux and Bryan Kane of Publicis, Canada for helping me with logistics of online publishing. Danish Siddiqui and Giuliano Magnoni helped me with all the electronic matters and the website. Thank you both. Finally, I thank my friend Ruggero Magnoni for his faith in my work and for all the support he gave me. Thank you all who believed in me and allowed me to prove my point.

Finally I am deeply grateful to His Majesty Sultan Qaboos Bin Said Al Said of The Sultanate of Oman and His Royal Highness The Prince of Wales, for continually supporting me and my work for almost two decades. Their patronage has been a constant source of encouragement.

Dr. Mosaraf Ali
February 2011

Dr. Ali's Books & Products:

The Integrated Health Bible | Women's Health Bible | Ultimate Back Book

Therapeutic Yoga | Weight Loss Plan | Nutrition Bible

- Detox Tea
  This is a blend of traditionally used herbs that helps to control excess stomach acid, suppress fungal and yeast overgrowth and restore functions of the liver. It is also used in Dr Ali's Detox Programme and Weight loss plan.

- Himalayan Tea
  It is a blend of White tea, holy basil, wild mint and Rhodedendron flowers collected at over 8000 ft by local villagers. Local people used it to prevent common ailments.

- Dr Ali's Joint and Bone Support:
  A blend of vitamins, minerals and supplements, that is useful for Joint and Bone care.

- Dr Ali's Women's Support:
  Natural supplements useful in maintaining women's general welbeing.

- Dr Ali's Immune Support:
  A blend of vitamins, minerals and supplements useful for maintaining the balance of The Immune System.

- Dr Ali's Energy Support:
  A blend of vitamins, minerals and supplements useful in boosting Energy.

- Dr Ali's Sinus Oil:
  A blend of natural oils, used traditionally, to keep the nasal tract and sinuses clear.

- Joint Oil:
  A blend of natural oils used traditionally to help inflammation of joints and muscles.

- Back Massage Oil:
  A blend of natural oils used traditionally to help in soothing backache, muscle ache an tendonitis.

- Lifestyle Massage Oil:
  A blend of natural oils used traditionally for regular massage to relax the body and the mind.

- Junior Massage Oil:
  A blend of natural oils used traditionally for regular massage of babies and children.

- Elixir Vita:
  A blend of natural tinctures, blended with fruit juices and used as a tonic to boost energy.(Contains alcohal)

- Elixir Nutrigest
  A tonic to aid digestion made from blended natural tinctures and fruit juices.
  (Contains alcohol)

- Elixir Tranquil :
  A blend of natural tinctures and floral extracts, used traditionally to relax the mind and body and aid sound sleep. (Contains alcohol)

To order these books & products email shop@integratedmed.co.uk